Carrie Schell

YOGA RECOVERY

A MIND-BODY-SPIRIT JOURNEY TO WELLNESS

AUSTIN MACAULEY PUBLISHERS™

LONDON • CAMBRIDGE • NEW YORK • SHARJAH

Ordering Information:
Quantity sales: special discounts are available on quantity purchases by corporations, associations, and others. For details, contact the publisher at the address below.

Publisher's cataloguing in publishing data
Schell, Carrie
Yoga Recovery: A Mind-Body-Spirit Journey to Wellness

ISBN 9781641827430 (Paperback)
ISBN 9781641827447 (Hardback)
ISBN 9781641827454 (E-Book)

The main category of the book — Health & Fitness / Yoga

www.austinmacauley.com/us

First Published (2019)
Austin Macauley Publishers LLC
40 Wall Street, 28th Floor
New York, NY 10005
USA

mail-usa@austinmacauley.com
+1 (646) 5125767

This book represents a culmination of years of thought, prayer, hard work, and determination. I wasn't clear how I should begin the book. In fact, there have been many variations; written and discarded. Inspiration finally came to me watching one of my teachers, Gabrielle Bernstein, during one of her Master Classes. In that moment, what to write became clear; to tell my authentic story, share with you what has called me to this moment, and share the intention of Mind Body Spirit.

Initially, I started off thinking I would share my story of growing-up in what I thought was a perfect family and how it all fell apart in the late 1970s with two tragedies that ended my fairy tale upbringing: my dad left our family and my aunt and five cousins died when their home caught on fire. This was the beginning of my life involving alcoholism and addiction. The twists and turns my life has taken are incredible. My head even spins thinking about it. Even though my story would make an incredibly juicy read, was that truly what I felt I needed to share? Sure, it would be entertaining and a page-turner, but was that my intention?

And, then, finally, on the morning of April 8th, listening to the teachings of Gabrielle Bernstein, I finally understood the real value in my story comes from my intention.

What is it that I truly feel moved to share? What is it that I would like to offer you? Through meditation and prayer, it became clear that my intention is to bring light to others so that they, so that you, may see and know the love and light within them. My intention for you is to know happiness and joy.

So, where is the real beginning?

Here Goes...

I believe I was called to serve early in my life. There has always been a voice calling me to God. I believe God is love. God is universal. God is everywhere and within everyone. God is the beauty in a sunset, the smile of stranger, and the love that exits.

The call, if you will, has manifested itself in my life at many times and in many ways.

When I say "serve", I mean be a voice of love. Be a light to others. Be a miracle worker. The wonderful text "Course in Miracles" describes a miracle as bringing love to others. This is what I mean by intention, when I speak about being called to serve.

There has always been a strong voice calling me to this. I know so many of us, most of us, are afraid to speak of such things. We worry people will think we've lost it, or they'll make assumptions about who we are, how we think, and live our lives. There are those who attribute close mindedness or a lack of enlightenment with those who speak of their spiritual life. To speak of God and love, and our spiritual life is foreign to us. For me, it is simple; God is Love! God is universal. God is everywhere and within everyone. That divine love is in us all, not just the chosen few. Isn't that an amazing gift? Love is everywhere and within everyone. I am no longer afraid to own my love for love! It is a gift I treasure. I hope with time you will allow yourself the opportunity to explore and own your spiritual pathway. As the wonderful teacher, Tommy Rosen, puts it, "Your spiritual path is the pathway to move and hear from the callings of your own heart."

In the Beginning...

I grew up in a Catholic family, going to church every Sunday and of course, dressed to perfection on the big days, Christmas and Easter. My family has a long and prominent history in the Catholic Church in Toronto, where I grew up. My family is huge, stereotypically, Catholic huge. My dad came from a family of 11 kids, I know, crazy! My mom has one brother and two sisters. Each of my mom's sisters had 11 kids and my uncle adopted seven. I'm not kidding! So, when I say my family is big, I mean it.

Our extended family was always very close when I grew up. Family played a huge role in shaping me. We always got together on holidays, weekends, Church on Sunday followed by breakfast and Saturday night, burgers at Nana and Papa's. But here's the funny thing. Even though I went to Catholic schools all of my life and went to Church, there was no talk of God, of God's love, or any sort of spiritual life in our home. Thinking back on it, Church was somewhere you went and followed rituals, but it had no impact on our day to day life. It was ritualistic and academic rather than spiritual and inspiring.

Being Catholic played a significant role in my life, but it had zero impact on my heart or spiritual life. Being Catholic was something you did by going to Church, celebrating First Communion, Confirmation, and of course, First Confession. Who can forget that? That kind of sums up my religious life growing up. Catholicism was part of my life, but it was a series of rituals and a source of confusion. I always longed for more. The memories I have filled with love, joy, and happiness came from time spent with my family and our huge extended family, not the Church. There was a true expression of love present in my childhood, but that came from my family and I sure didn't associate it with God.

I can remember experiencing feelings of great love while in church. But this love came with the need to keep a close reign over my emotions; I felt that if I were to truly let go, let in the love of God I was experiencing, I would be overwhelmed and called to action. I felt I would need to live my life spreading light and love. At that time, I believed that I would have to sacrifice all of the normal experiences of being a teenager to answer the call. I had visions of the nuns who taught me in school. As a teenager, all I knew was that I longed for travel, adventure, experiences, and love. Those longings didn't fit in with my limited understanding of what being spiritual was all about. I did know I didn't want to be a nun, so I ignored the calling.

When I was in my early twenties, I had already spent summers backpacking through Europe, traveling, and living in France while going to university. It was at this time that voice within me, my Inner Guide, my Spirit began to call me again. And this time, I began to listen. This time I began to let my light shine on others.

It was then that I began to experience a true selfless love for others, when I was touring around as a Deadhead. I experienced this love through sharing music, food, and song with others who also longed for a sense of community, love, and belonging. My friends and I were all wanting to tap into a greater source of love and spread that love to others. At the time, this was the only way we knew how to live a spiritual life of love and sharing.

It was during this time that I met the Community, a group of people who would travel to the Dead shows; speaking of love and God. I was drawn to their spiritual life, their communal way of living, and how they reached out to others. My relationship with the Community grew, leading me to eventually live with them in Vermont. I think my family thought I was absolutely insane. I gave away all of my worldly possessions; not much at the time and off I went, to live in the Community! It was very much a commune-type of life. We all worked together and lived in these incredible Victorian homes. We ate together, played music and worshiped, and prayed as one. To many peoples' surprise, there was no drinking or drugs in life at the Community. I remember feeling so peaceful there, so content. I remember reading scripture and having it finally make sense in the context I was living. This is what it means to love your neighbour and they were living it daily!

Of course, I was in my twenties and when my boyfriend left the Community, I was only weeks behind choosing to leave the life of love, peace, and simplicity I had found to be with him. Ah, of course, there was the boyfriend. We had gone to the Community together, searching. Afterward, I remember wondering if I had made an incredible mistake in leaving to be with him. Would I be able to experience that sense of community again? I had always wanted to go back, to experience that sense of true community and fellowship. People living to love and support one another. But it just wasn't to be. As much as I loved being there, I somehow knew there were things I needed to do within the world that kept me from returning.

A couple of years passed and I found myself sitting, listening to Ina May Gaskin, the founder of modern midwifery and author of *Spiritual Midwifery,* giving a talk at Dalhousie University in Halifax, Canada. It was as if the "ah hah!" light went off. In that instant, I knew I was called to be a midwife. Before that talk, I can honestly say that I don't think I had even heard the term midwife. Midwifery had not experienced the resurgence and legitimization that it experiences today. Midwives were few and far between, and most definitely, not part of the health care system. As for education, the apprenticeship model was still largely the only way to become a midwife; a stark contrast from today's career option and university education!

And so Ina May became my first teacher of midwifery. It was on her recommendation that I found myself living in El Paso, Texas attending Maternidad la Luz, learning from two of the most incredible women and midwives I have been blessed to meet, Deborah Kaley and Diane Alcorn. To be a midwife at that time was more than a profession, it was a spiritual calling. You had to be extremely committed to being a midwife. Back then a midwife was always needing to legitimize her practice, skills, and education. And it didn't exactly pay. In fact, I rarely got paid for the care I provided. I did get some nice chickens, an out of tune piano, and lots of heart-felt love and gratitude for guiding a soul into the world, an exchange more valuable than money. The joy I felt, helping women throughout her pregnancy year is hard to express. Helping a woman through one of the most sacred journeys she will ever experience with dignity, respect, and love cannot be matched. Having the honour of bringing a new spirit into the world in a safe and loving environment is such a gift I was blessed to share. I love being a midwife. It is part of who I am and continues to shape the person I am.

But the call did not end there. It is truly incredible how when the universe closes a door, it always opens a window!

I was beginning to stagnate in my midwifery career. I had gone as far as I could in Nova Scotia. I was the President of the provincial association and had spent countless years lobbying government for the legalization and regulation of midwives. Unfortunately, the victory of legislation had a cost; it made the midwives cutthroat and bureaucratic. I had had enough. I needed a change, but wasn't sure where that change was leading me. The spirit and heart of midwifery had become jaded in the fight for power and I wanted out.

I began looking at what options were available to me. I did a Master's degree, I felt it would give me the knowledge and credibility to take my career further in health and wellness. Realizing this wasn't the solution I was seeking, I felt moved to become a doctor. I then began working away on my Science degree. Convinced this was the path I should be on, I applied to medical school and was accepted. And so, one August, I moved to the West Indies to attend medical school, away from my husband and children, the youngest being two at the time. When I look back on it, what was I thinking? I had been confident that our marriage and family were strong enough to endure the separation, but the exact opposite was true.

Medical school lasted only one semester. The challenge was too great for my family and the realities of life brought me back to my home to Canada. I was devastated when that door closed and it would take me months to emerge from the sadness of knowing I would not be a doctor. It took even longer to replace those feelings of loss with a deep gratitude for the gift of my family. The door to medical school may have closed and that dream ended, but I had the greater joy, love, and gratitude for my family. If that door hadn't closed, I would not have the deep loving relationship I do with my children. I wouldn't know them. That closing door blessed me with the awareness and understanding that being a mom;

sharing a deep love with my children is my greatest joy! It is amazing how with time we understand the blessings given to us. Time allows us to see the grace the universe has bestowed upon us.

At this point in time, I didn't know what to do! I lived in a very rural community in Nova Scotia, where opportunities, which were of interest to me and in keeping with my education and experience, were not to be found within 200 km. I began a PhD and hoped something would manifest itself. Part of me still believed that my worth and value were somehow dependent on my career and earnings.

In the meantime, since I couldn't make use of my education and years' experience, I thought I would focus on doing something I loved – physical activity.

Throughout my life as a mom (maybe a good time to mention that I have seven children), I realized that a key to my mental wellness and happiness was physical activity. At first, when I began running; it was a slow and grueling process. It wasn't a pretty site when I first started running or what I refer to as "moving my legs in rapid succession." But with time and perseverance, I actually began to love and hate running. To be fair to myself, I became quite a good runner, but it was never effortless. I would hear people talk about getting into a groove and being able to run forever. That wasn't me. Each run was a fight to the finish. When my kids were babies, I would run inside on our treadmill. As soon as the baby (which ever one was the baby at the time) was having a nap, I would zip on that thing and run five km. Wham! Done and my sanity restored. I saw the connection, immediately. The connection was so clear not only to me but to others that when I would get grumpy or bitchy, my husband would "encourage" me to go for a run. No lie!

I began to look for ways to turn my love for the outdoors and physical activity into my livelihood. So, I became a certified personal trainer, fitness instructor, and group cardio instructor. I never had any intention of being a trainer or instructing classes, I just like pushing myself and this was a good way to do it. I hoped it would eventually lead me to what I was to do in life.

It was with this new set of skills and certifications, combined with my previous health background that I somehow ended up as the Director of Health and Wellness at a 30 day residential addiction centre that was going to be opening in the area. Because it was a new facility, I had *carte blanche* to design the health and wellness program. It was an incredibly scary opportunity, but very exciting. It was here that the seeds of mind, body, and spirit were planted.

I developed a program that was rooted in daily yoga, guided meditation, and physical activity. I also led the clients in a cognitive-behavioural session daily. I would take the clients out on hikes to the ocean; meditating, reflecting, and sharing, overlooking the beauty of the waves. The positive impact this was having on the clients was immediately evident. The combination of yoga, physical activity, and meditation allowed clients to reconnect with their inner Self, their true Self. The reconnecting with the Self was a powerful experience to witness and share, and the key to their success in the program.

This was an exciting time, but I have to admit that I was pretty conflicted about working at the centre. I had spent years, decades even, trying to eliminate alcoholism and addiction from my life, and now, I was working six days a week with people in recovery. I kept asking God why alcohol and drugs were always playing such a significant role in my life, both; personally and professionally. I just wanted them gone and now I was completely immersed in that world.

It is amazing how when you put your needs out there to the universe and are willing to listen, you will get an answer.

My answer arrived when a client in recovery said to me, "You see me, the real me." That was it, it all made sense and became crystal clear! The years of addiction and alcoholism in my life had gifted me with the ability to see through the substance use, to see the real person, and the light within them. In that instant, I knew I was in the right place in the right moment. It all started making sense. The connections were becoming clear. The same calling that had led me to become a midwife; to share the most intimate and vulnerable time in a woman's life was the same call that was leading me to shine the light of love on someone in their intimate and vulnerable time of recovery. In every client who came to the centre, I could see their true self, the inner child, the inner divine, whatever name you want to call it. It was that inner spirit, that light, that I would help ignite within each client. I then began to notice how connecting with ones' physical self through yoga or a hike, or mediation at the ocean was often the gateway to connecting with the true self. These tiny connections would grow and rekindle a sense of self-esteem and self-worth within the clients.

But here's the kicker; even though I could find peace and love through the chaos of alcoholism and addiction with others, I still agonized over the role alcoholism and addiction were playing in my personal life. I still prayed for it to be gone away from me. It was great helping others through recovery, but I sure as hell didn't want to have to deal with it in my personal life. And yet, there it was. I couldn't escape it. Alcoholism and addiction continued to follow to me.

I am continually amazed how the universe hears our prayers. The thing is, the answers come in their time, in their way. And guess what? The universe's timings and solutions always serve us best. At the time, I was growing impatient and frustrated. I was ready to give up and abandon hope. But the universe knows. I always think of the saying, "God only gives us what we can handle." That has often come to mind and I have thought *Wow! God must think I am Wonder Woman! And you know what? Even when my life seemed absolutely crazy, like there could not be one more thing that I could endure, I realized the truth in that saying. I am Wonder Woman! I can endure. I am strong.* And so, I continued on, not understanding why my life was immersed, both, personally and professionally in alcoholism and addiction, even though I longed to escape it.

And then, tiny miracles began to happen. Out of the depths of despair, when I was feeling beaten, that I was not that wonder woman, God kept telling me I was, miracles were born! Miracles are those tiny glimmers of love we witness and share.

And because of miracles, I am now fearless! There is no fear in the light of love. I see that I am called to jump into alcoholism and addiction; this is where I am supposed to be. My strengths and talents have brought me to where I am meant to be; serving people who need love and compassion during this part of their journey. I now see that my sense of worth and purpose comes from being of service to others. My journey involves bringing together my passions and my strengths, and sharing them. There is a reason alcoholism and addiction have been part of my life for such a long time. It has given me the tools and compassion I need to be doing the work I am meant to be doing. The Call I have always heard, is the call to share the miracles, the universe, God; that love has to offer and bring hope, and love to others. It is the call to say, "I see you! I hear you! You are worthy!"

I promise you that when you let the light in, miracles will happen! You will experience forgiveness and love. You will see the true you, once again. You will fall in love with all that you are! You are perfection! Past all that you perceive are your failings and shortcomings is the real you; the you that radiates love to others, when you allow the true self to shine.

It is through yoga, meditation, and physical activity that you will cultivate that relationship with your true self, the self beyond the addiction and alcoholism, the self beyond the disappointments and perceived failures. You are stronger than you know! God only sends you that which you can handle. The fact that you are here today; that you have endured alcoholism and addiction, despite the odds, is a miracle! You have a purpose. Your work here is not finished, it is just beginning! I want you to take a moment and think about that, let it sink in. Beyond all odds, you are here, alive. You are given another opportunity to live the life you were meant to live! How friggin' amazing is that? You have work to do! It is not luck or coincidence that you are coming out on the other side of alcoholism and addiction. You are stronger than you know. You are here for a purpose. Take that in! That, in itself, is a miracle!

I do not think words can convey how blessed I feel to be part of the journey that you are on. The strength and courage that you have is mind-blowing. Only others who have traveled the road of recovery, can appreciate the strength and will power it takes. I am honoured to be sharing that journey with you. I do not say that lightly. I say that from the heart of one who has had alcohol and addiction play a central role in her life for decades in various forms. I want to share with you, with all my heart, that you can live a happy (and for me, happy is not some trite word to be thrown out there. It has true value. It is our purpose in life!) joyful life, where you find love for yourself, first and foremost, and love for others. I don't mean to minimize the challenges being sober presents, but I do mean to offer hope! I do offer a promise. You are here, reading this for a reason. Believe. Hang in there!

You can do this! I am with you. All of the love of the universe is with you. Let it in. Remember, it is no coincidence that you are here, getting sober. You are not done, you are meant to do great things. Trust and believe in the power of love!

It is my hope to shine the light on your body, mind, and spirit, allowing you to develop a deep relationship with all that you are. You are light, love, peace, joy, and happiness. Trust in miracles and love.

Love

I wanted to take a moment to thank you for the courageous journey that you are on. I know how challenging it can be, the struggles, the worries, the self-doubt. But the fact that you are here today, reading this, ready to do yoga is absolutely inspiring to me. I want to thank you with such gratitude for continuing on. Know that you are worth it. Know that days will get better. This will get easier.

In order for us to truly understand the root of our addiction, it's important to begin to identify our emotions. For simplicity's sake, we can think in general terms of negative and positive emotions. We need to begin to be able to identify our negative emotions that don't bring us happiness, peace or joy, silence or contentment. There are a million labels for negative emotions: jealousy, anger, hate, fear, depression, greed, envy, despair, stress, anxiety. Any emotions and feelings that don't provide us with a sense of security and love, are ones that we really need to be mindful of. When we find we are experiencing the negative, we need to learn to pause, take a moment before we speak, before we act, and just, really acknowledge the true place our feelings are coming from. Most of our negative emotions come from a place of fear, a lack of love of some sort; fear of lack, fear of insecurity, fear of self-worthlessness, or fear of low self-esteem. When we are in this place of fear, it is almost impossible to experience love and happiness. We must learn to begin to cultivate actions and thoughts that keep us in the positive; nurturing love within us. It is when we are able to release our negative emotions and fears that we are able to reach our highest potential rooted in love.

It is also important to know that a life of sobriety does not mean that we won't have struggles, challenges, and doubts. But with time and mindfulness set on love and happiness, it will not be a life that is ruled by the negative. With time, it will become a life where we are not ruled by negative emotions and actions. We will begin to experience a life rooted in love with a full range of emotions, feelings, and thoughts; positive and negative. And in time, when we experience negative thoughts and feelings, we will be able to take a moment and reflect, and really let them go. And I believe at the heart letting go is forgiveness.

Forgiveness, ultimately, is built upon the foundation of love. We cannot totally forgive someone unless we love. And that love doesn't start with loving someone else; it starts with loving the self. And I know that is hard to take in, it is hard to swallow and comprehend because for most of us, we are not brought up that way. We are not brought up to think of loving the self; we are brought up to think of loving others. Most of us feel uncomfortable, boastful, conceited, negative words and attachments associated with the most incredible, necessary, positive emotion; loving one's self.

It is not out of conceit, or lack of humility, or lack of grace that we love ourselves.

Loving one's self is acknowledging the Divine in this world that we are part of. The Divine is in us. It is part of everything around us. It is part of the crocuses coming up in the spring. It is in the miracle of a salmon returning to spawn where it was born, year after year as it makes the arduous journey up the falls, through the streams. It is in the miracle of nature, in the beauty of our world. We are part of that, we are not separate. God, the Divine, wants us to see and know that. God wants us to open our eyes and say *Wow! I have been so wrong! I have been thinking I need to protect myself and wear my armor in order to be good or strong in all that this world recognizes!* When really, we need to be able to say *I love me! The fact that I am here makes me of such value and of such worth.*

When we can really love ourselves and stop the self-criticism and self-judgments, love enters and forgiveness begins. Instead of being bound by negative emotions, we are able to forgive ourselves and in doing so, forgive others. The more we forgive others, the more we experience forgiveness ourselves. It is such a beautiful cyclical experience.

I experience this powerful exchange when I am able to look at my teenage son, who has been a source of frustration and challenge. I look at him with a love that melts him and lets him know, "You are my son. I love you. There is nothing we cannot do. And you are nothing but greatness." The softness and love he shows me in return is such a gift; this gift is a miracle. The miracle ends the cycle of strife and conflict, and replaces it with one of grace and love. Believe me, my son can still be a challenge, but I am able to approach him with love. It doesn't mean that we don't have to work at our relationship. We need to mindful of our actions and their impact on ourselves and others. We need to surround ourselves with positive, nurturing, loving energy to feed our heart and mind. It does require effort and mindfulness. It is challenging to let judgments, sarcasm, and negativity go. But, when you do, it is so worth it!

So, don't be discouraged when you are feeling the negative. We are human with a full range of emotions. Sometimes through experiences of sadness, anger, and despair, we come to know what great happiness, joy, and kindness are. I am encouraging you to acknowledge the negative and take a moment before you react and use words, or act in ways that may cause harm. When our words cause harm, we often find ourselves needing to take a righteous attitude to defend our behaviour. This only creates another layer between our self and happiness.

Happiness is our purpose in life. The way to happiness is through forgiveness. The way to forgiveness is love. And how wonderful is it to know that we can easily live in that world of love! How blessed are we. How miraculous is it that we've been living in this world where we have been running around crazy, doing all of these horrible things to ourselves mentally, physically, and spiritually, which can all be undone! The craziness and fear can be undone in the blink of an eye. You are so worthy! When you begin to share your love and let that light shine on others, it will allow the light and love of others to shine. That is the cycle we want to be a part of. We want to live in that cycle. We want to step into the cycle of happiness, love, and forgiveness and out of the cycle of the fear, pain, and negativity.

So, what if everything we thought about addiction was wrong?

Maybe We've Got It All Wrong…

The importance of human connections and bonding is the topic of Johann Hari's Ted Talk from 2015, which challenges that almost everything we thought about addictions is wrong. If you aren't familiar with the Talk, check it out; it's quite amazing. I want to share with you a snapshot of his game-changing talk.

Johann begins the talk exploring the notion of addiction being caused by chemical hooks in drugs. Here is how he began to understand addictions differently.

Bruce Alexander, professor of psychology, at Simon Fraser University in Vancouver, noted that most of our ideas of chemical hooks emerged largely from rat experiments in the 20th century. In the experiments, isolated rats were put in cages with two water bottles; one with cocaine or heroin water and the other bottle only had water. Almost always, the rats preferred the drug water and almost always killed themselves quite quickly.

In the 1970's, Alexander was looking at the experiment and said, "We've got a rat in an empty cage. Let's try something." And that something, is what Alexander called Rat Park. Rather than being put alone in empty cage, Rat Park had tunnels, rat wheels, food, companions to interact and have sex with, and loads of stimuli. He also put both types of water as in the original experiment.

Here's the thing; the rats didn't like the drug water, they almost never used it. None of them used it compulsively and none of them ever overdosed.

So, you go from almost 100% overdose when they are isolated, to 0% when they have happy and connected lives.

Initially, Professor Alexander wondered if this could be specific to rat behaviour. Interestingly, at the same time, there was a real life human example being lived out – the Vietnam War.

In Vietnam, 20% of all US troops were heavily using heroin. There was fear this would result in hundreds of thousands of junkies in the United States when the soldiers returned home.

When the heroin using soldiers returned home, they were followed in a study published in the Archives of General Psychiatry and this is what they found:

The soldiers didn't enter rehab. They didn't go into withdrawal. 95% of them just stopped. 95! This brings into question the chemical hook theory.

Professor Alexander began to wonder if there was a different story to addiction. What if addiction is not simply about chemical hooks, but about your cage – your adaptation to your environment. And other academics began to look at this.

Peter Cohen, a professor in the Netherlands, proposed, "Maybe we shouldn't even call it addiction, maybe we should call it bonding."

This Is Where It Gets Interesting...

Cohen states humans have a natural and innate need to bond. When we are happy and healthy, we bond and connect with each other. He further states that if you cannot do that, you can't bond, because you are traumatized, isolated, or beaten down by life, struggling with mental illness, or whatever the cause – you will bond with something that will give you some sense of relief. That something can be drugs, alcohol, sex, eating, shopping, gambling, pornography, your cellphone, but you will bond and connect with something because that is in our nature.

When you are happy and thriving in your life, you have bonds and connections you want to be present, for that keep you from being an addict or alcoholic, even though you have the opportunity to become one. You have people you love, including yourself. You have a sense of purpose and happy relationships.

Through this lens, disconnection with others and a lack of bonds is a major driver of addiction.

There's more...

Environmental writer, Bill McKibben, in an article originally published in *Speaking Truth to Power* theorizes why Americans are so lonely. He points out that the number of close friends the average American feels they can count on in a crisis has been steadily declining since the 1950s. Interestingly, during the same time period, the amount of floor space an individual has in their home has been steadily increasing.

He suggests it's a metaphor for our culture: We've traded floor space for friends, we've traded things for connections and the result is we are one of the loneliest societies there has ever been. We are creating our own cage, moving away from our relationships and connections to a life of isolation.

So, what does this all really mean and what is the connection with yoga?

I think, if we are really candid, it is hard loving an addict or alcoholic and perhaps, it's even more difficult loving yourself as the alcoholic or addict.

We have so many messages about how to respond to addicts – just say no, or maybe we distance ourselves and walk away, we have interventions and tough love ultimatums. But what this is really doing, is taking the already fragile connections and bonds in the addict's life and threatening them. Threatening the thing they long for and need.

Really, we should be looking for ways to strengthen and nurture those bonds. We need to find ways to deepen the connections in our relationships with the alcoholics and addicts we care for and to also help deepen the connections, and love they have for themselves.

And this is where yoga comes in – beyond the physical practice and straight to the heart.

My Yoga Journey

When I began to practice yoga, for me, it was a completely physical thing. It was a fitness thing that I was including as part of my work out schedule. I practiced yoga at home, alone. I began doing yoga when my husband suggested we start doing P90X; an intense 90 day program that included yoga on its rest day. And so, I came to yoga through P90X, through a very physical and competitive push yourself program. I loved the physical, asana practice of yoga. I clearly remember saying to myself, "I am never getting into the whole spiritual side of yoga!" I was not getting into the whole yoga scene. I had done the whole commune, hippy thing. For me, it was a physical practice, a physical thing. I enjoyed pushing myself and yoga was a new challenge, nothing more. I was adamant that yoga would always be about fitness for me. I swore I would never learn Sanskrit or pick up a book on yoga. No ohms, meditation, or chanting. I was very determined and clear that this was not part of what yoga was for me, this was just a workout.

The longer I stuck with yoga, the more I began thinking about becoming an instructor. I think it appealed to my competitive nature. Even though I had no intention of teaching yoga at this point, I wanted to have the feeling of mastery. I've always liked the idea of mastering things. So, the next natural progression, for me, was to become a yoga instructor. Living 200 kilometers from the nearest yoga class, the only way I could become a yoga instructor was through a fitness company that offered yoga instructor certification. At the time, the course really appealed to me because it was pretty much all physical and no spiritual stuff. So, I did the first level, which allowed me to instruct. I was a yoga instructor, kind of...

Around six months after doing the yoga instructor course, a dear friend, Eoin Finn, was in town. I hadn't seen Eoin in way too many years. He was in Halifax leading a yoga workshop for Lu Lu Lemon and I was there doing my second yoga instructor level. We hadn't seen each other for over twenty years and now, after all this time, we were in the same city for yoga. It was the perfect chance to get together and connect. When we were in university, we were really close. We were really blessed with a great community of friends back then and we had some amazing experiences together. We were on our spiritual journey even back then, searching through friends, music, celebration, and nature.

So, Eoin was in town and we were trying to get together for a coffee. I can remember that when we got together I had this kind of shameful feeling when we met. I wouldn't understand why I was feeling that way for quite some time after seeing him. You see, Eoin is an incredible yogi, he embodies the spirit of yoga and it radiates from within. He has the light and that light shines in him! I remember feeling so fraudulent. I was on this path of becoming a "yoga teacher" when I didn't embrace yoga. It was so great to see him, but something wasn't right. It's not that we were talking about the spiritual practice of yoga, or having this deeply spiritual conversation, but it was just something… Being in his presence, I realized I couldn't continue on the path of yoga training I was on. It was seeing in him that I realized that the way I was going about my instructor training was not complete. I respected yoga enough at the time to see that there was beauty in yoga beyond the physical practice, if I was willing to commit to it. Because of that encounter, I knew that if I wasn't going to do the full meal deal and cultivate a mind, body, spirit approach to my yoga practice, I shouldn't be an instructor. The training I was receiving was very physical and skimmed the surface of yoga, not the heart of yoga, that much I knew.

Although I didn't realize it at the time, that was the start of my true love for yoga. Not for the physical practice, but for yoga in its entirety. It was a beautiful moment when I came to that realization that the beauty of yoga is far greater than the physical asana practice. In that meeting with Eoin, I realized that I was not honouring yoga with all it required. I knew in that moment I felt embarrassed. Why was I feeling that way? Why was I embarrassed? I had been clear I had just only wanted a physical practice of yoga, so why the embarrassment?

I think in that moment when I met with Eoin, I saw what truly embracing and fully living yoga was. My heart stirred…something had been awakened in me.

The beauty is, that from that experience I went on to do my yoga teacher training a couple of years later and this time, it was the real deal. This time, I felt that blessed to go. And here's the whole 180 thing. When I went to do my yoga training at Yandara in Baja, I didn't go for the physical mastery or becoming a yoga instructor. I went because I knew I needed a spiritual reawakening. I knew my spirit was struggling. I was at a low point in my life that was so challenging. I knew I needed something. This time, my main objective in my yoga journey was to have my spirit healed. It overwhelms me to even think of that time. I was blessed for the journey. I was blessed that I came away from that journey with new understandings and learnings that still continue to unfold and grow. My incredible teacher, Christopher Perkins, guided me gently into the heart of yoga and let me take in its love.

I was blessed to realize and understand that the universe has divine timing. It sets you up with where you need to go. It was because of the spiritual reawakening I experienced during my yoga journey, I realized that all of the other professional work I was doing at the time, valuable in its own right, was not spiritually fulfilling. My work had been focused on increasing the health of our children and youth through physical activity. We live in such a sedentary, screen-based world that our children are suffering physically, emotionally, and mentally. I want "our" children to be healthy, full of vitality, and joy. I was developing valuable programs to increase the health of our children, but I suddenly realized that I was longing for the heart connection, for the spirit connection in my work again. I had that connection in my work as a midwife and my work at the addictions centre and I longed for it.

And so the 180 I experienced, from a mindset that yoga would always be a physical practice to a mindset that embraces yoga as the foundation of my spiritual journey is wow! As I am retelling this, I am in my car, speaking into a little recorder I keep with me. The sun is glowing, guiding my drive. So, yes! Thank you! Thank you, God! Thank you to the Divine within me! Thank you, Universe! I have such gratitude. I trust and believe in the power of love. Thank you for being here with me. We will be on this journey together! This is the beginning of your physical and spiritual yoga practice; created for you from a place of love, blessings, and gratitude.

Namaste.

Thank You!

Thank you! Thank you for having the strength and courage to open this book. The last 38 years of my life have been shaped by alcoholism and addiction. The fact that you are here on this journey, signals hope and love! It is my intention that *Mind, Body, Spirit* be a light in your day, a light that will shine on your true Self, that source of love and goodness. Be kind to yourself. Never lose sight of the truth that you are here, in this moment, reading this with every intention of living a life of clarity and purpose. You may stumble and lose your way, but please do not give up. You are worthy of all of the love and goodness divinely present! I am sending you love and blessings through *Mind, Body, Spirit* to help carry you. Thank you for being you! Thank you for being present and having the courage to continue your journey. You have my deepest admiration and respect. Namaste!

I promise you, that when you let the light in miracles will happen! You will experience forgiveness and love. You will see the true you once again and fall in love with you! You are perfection! Past all what you perceive are your failings and shortcomings, it is you that radiates love to others when you allow the true Self to shine.

Happiness Explained

Happiness is the meaning and the purpose of life, the whole aim, and end of human experience.

– Aristotle

The word happy seems to have lost its meaning today. It's kind of like the word 'nice'. We use it as a general catch all. But do we truly understand what genuine happiness is and the significant impact it can have on our lives? Happiness is a state of being free from fear, anger, attack, and hate. Happiness is the state in which we were created. I would even go so far to say that being happy, truly happy, is not only our responsibility, but our right.

What is happiness and how can we attain it?

Happiness is the overall experience of pleasure and meaning. Happy people enjoy positive emotions while knowing their life as purposeful, with meaning. Happiness comes not from a single moment, but from the overall state of being one is in. A person can endure emotional pain at times and still be happy overall.

Believe it or not, there have even been studies that show there is a direct relationship between happiness and success. Not only can success – in work, sobriety or in love – contribute to happiness, but happiness also leads to more success. So what does that mean? Everything being equal, happy people have better relationships. They are more likely to thrive at work and also, live better, and longer. Happiness is a worthwhile pursuit, whether as an end in itself or as a way to be "successful" in other aspects of your life.

Don't ask yourself what the world needs; ask yourself what makes you come alive. And then, go and do that. Because what the world needs, is people who have come alive.

– Harold Whitman

Happiness Is Key...

The idea that our actions should be guided by self-interest, by or own happiness, is important. I'm not suggesting that we be self-absorbed and out only for ourselves. When we begin to live our lives in a way that is truly happy, it brings meaning and what is really cool is that it has an overflow effect on others. Our happiness is contagious. That's why helping others is so important in creating a happy life. Of course, it's important to keep in mind the difference between helping others and living for other's happiness. If we don't make the pursuit of our own happiness a priority, we are denying our true Self. An unhappy person is less likely to be benevolent, and that leads to further unhappiness. When we're happy, we are more likely to see beyond our narrow, inward-looking, and self-centred perspective and focus on other's needs and wants.

When we make choices, we first need to ask ourselves what would make us happy, regardless of how much it might add to the happiness of others. We also need to ask ourselves whether what we want to do would deprive someone else of their own happiness, because this would take away from our own happiness.

Happiness is not about sacrifice or a trade-off between present and future benefit, between meaning and pleasure or between helping only ourselves and helping others. It is about balance; about creating a life in which all of these elements, which are essential to happiness, are in harmony.

Most people are about as happy as they make up their minds to be.

– Abraham Lincoln

Why would anyone actively deprive himself of happiness? In her book *A Return to Love* Marianne Williamson says:

"Our deepest fear is not that we are inadequate. Our deepest fear is that we are powerful beyond measure. It is our light, not our darkness, that most frightens us. We ask ourselves who am I to be brilliant, beautiful, talented, and amazing? Actually, who are you not to be?"

Why are we not being happy? Why does the light frighten us more than the dark? Why do we think that we are unworthy of happiness?

There are external and internal factors, cultural and psychological biases that work against us being happy. On the most fundamental level, the idea that we have the right to be happy, that individual happiness is a noble and worthy pursuit, isn't something most of us are brought up believing.

Many of us have limitations that are self-generated; that we create ourselves. When we do not feel that we are worthy of happiness, we can't possibly feel worthy of the good things in our lives; the things that bring us happiness, because we don't believe we actually deserve them. Happiness really could be ours, but we deny ourselves the opportunity to attain it. This creates behaviours which lead to a self-fulfilling prophecy: we are not worthy of happiness and so we don't work towards that which makes us happy, in turn, bringing us more unhappiness.

Even if we do find happiness, we might feel guilty because there are other people who are less fortunate. We feel there is a finite amount of happiness, love, and abundance in this world. We even feel that one person's happiness (ours included) will deprive others of theirs. The truth is far from this. When we let our light shine, we unconsciously give other people permission to do the same.

Inherent Worthiness

To lead a happy life, we must experience a sense of inherent worthiness. Okay, what do I mean by this? Inherent worthiness is the value we have, simply because we were born, because we are here. In order to seek joy and happiness, a person must first believe they are worthy of having them. In order to fight for happiness, we must consider ourselves worthy of happiness. We must appreciate our core self, our true Self, who we really are beyond our accomplishments. We must believe that we deserve to be happy. We must feel that we are worthy, by virtue of our existence, because we were born with a heart and mind to experience pleasure and meaning of true happiness.

When we don't accept our inherent worth, we ignore and actively undermine our talents, our potential, our joy, our accomplishments. Okay, for example, we might have the "yes, but…" approach. "Yes, I do have some meaning and pleasure in my life, but what if I doesn't last?" "Yes, I have found a partner I love, but what if they leave me?" "Yes, I love my job, but what if I get bored, like I usually do?" Refusing to accept the good things that happen to you and failure to recognize the good while you are experiencing it, leads to unhappiness.

So, how do we find happiness in our lives? How do we cultivate happiness?

Happiness is not some fleeting thing. There is so much we can do in our lives to develop a deep sense of happiness. It begins with believing in ourselves and developing our sense of worth, and self-esteem. It is only then, we can begin to align our lives with actions and emotions that bring us both, pleasure and meaning.

Pleasure and Meaning

Pleasure is about the experience of positive emotions in the here and now, it is about present benefit. Meaning comes from having a sense of purpose, from the lasting, positive future benefit of our actions.

Emotion, of course, plays an important role in all we do. Emotions cause motion; they provide motivation that drives our actions. What do I mean by that? Emotions motivate us to act and do things we want or desire. They can move us away from something we don't want; a desire-less state, providing us motivation to act in order to make things better. If we were free of emotion and its motivation to act, we would aspire to nothing. We would remain indifferent to our actions and thoughts as well as their ramifications. Because emotion is the foundation of motivation, it naturally plays a central role in us wanting to pursue happiness.

To be happy, we need the experience of positive emotions, so it only makes sense that pleasure is a part of what is needed for a fulfilling life.

Let's be clear, though. Please don't think that pleasure is about being in a state of ecstasy or being buzzed, or on a constant "high". We all experience emotional highs and lows. We can experience sadness at times – when we suffer a loss or failure – and still lead a happy life. In fact, the unrealistic expectation of a constant high, just leads to disappointment and feelings of inadequacy, and leads to negative emotions. It can also lead to the need to detach from the negative things in our lives through substances and alcohol.

Don't get me wrong, happy people experience highs and lows, but their overall state of being is positive. To be happy, we have to feel that whatever sorrows, trials, and tribulations we may encounter, we still experience the joy of being alive.

Is experiencing positive emotions all we need to be happy? When we experience emotions, we need to know that the feelings are real. This is important. The effect of drugs; especially, ecstasy inducing drugs feel good but they aren't real. You need to be truly present to know your emotional experiences are the real deal. Being happy then, is more than positive emotions; artificial or otherwise. We need more than the present sensation that we feel – we need the cause of our emotions to be meaningful. We want to know that our actions have an actual positive effect on our lives and in the world. We want to know that our experiences are not just fleeting emotions or feelings. We know our experiences have meaning because we have the capacity to reflect on our feelings, thoughts, and actions. We have the capacity to be aware of our consciousness and our experiences.

We also have the capacity for spirituality. The Oxford English Dictionary defines spirituality as, "the real sense of significance of something." When we speak of a meaningful life, we often talk of having a sense of purpose, but what we sometimes fail to recognize is that finding this sense of purpose means more than experiencing pleasure or setting goals. Having goals or even reaching them does not guarantee that we are leading a purposeful existence. To experience a sense of purpose, the goals we set for ourselves need to be fundamentally meaningful.

To live a meaningful life, we must have a self-generated purpose that has personal significance, rather than feeling we need to act and live in a way we feel is imposed upon us by family or society's standards and expectations. When we are able to do things which have true meaning for us, we begin to experience a sense of purpose. Sometimes, this purpose can hold such meaning for us that we feel as though we have found our calling. For me, being here for you is a calling – it is a meaningful career and spiritual journey dedicated to helping others.

Idealism and Realism

Being an idealist is being a realist in the deepest sense – it is being true to our real nature, our higher self. Without a higher purpose, a calling, or an ideal, we cannot reach our full potential for happiness. Being an idealist is about having a sense of purpose that our life is meaningful. We need to find meaning in our daily lives. So, let's say we have a sense of purpose in creating a happy family, we also need specific, attainable, day to day goals such as having dinner with our children or partner each evening. This sounds simple, but it is important because it can be difficult to sustain the big picture goals without being able to actualize them on the day to day level, which gives meaning to the present and short-term future. It's tough thinking about a life of sobriety when getting through the day without a drink is challenging. That's why it is key to go day by day. Celebrate each moment!

Potential and Happiness

When we think about creating a meaningful life for ourselves, it's really important to keep in mind our potential. What are our talents, skills, and gifts? How can we build upon and strengthen these to reach our full potential? It's one thing to do things that feel good in the moment, it's a whole other thing to do things that feel good while developing our potential. Take some time to think about things you love doing – things that serve you positively or things you're good at. How can you put your energy into those parts of your life to help you strive to meet your fullest potential in all areas of your life physically, emotionally and spiritually?

The Need for Meaning and Pleasure

Seeking pleasure is not enough to be happy. On the other hand, having only a sense of purpose will not bring us true meaning in our lives. We need both to experience true happiness. We need to experience both, purpose and positive emotions, to create meaning in our lives for the present and the future. We need to have the will for pleasure and the will for meaning, if we are going to lead a fulfilling, happy life. Having that will to pursue a life of happiness, love, and purpose is crucial; especially, when we are struggling to find meaning in our lives once our substance has been removed from the equation.

It's so important to remember that going through difficult times gives us the gift to appreciate pleasure. I know that's confusing, but it's true. Enduring challenges keeps us from taking pleasure for granted and it reminds us to be grateful for all of the small and large pleasures in our lives. Being grateful in this way, is actually a source of real meaning and pleasure.

There's a definite relationship between pleasure and meaning and between present and future benefit. When we get sense of purpose from what we do, our sense of pleasure is intensified. And when we feel good in what we're doing, it makes the experience all the more meaningful.

We rarely take time to reflect on whether or not the things we devote our time to actually bring us happiness. A great exercise is to take a moment and make a list of the things that you spend your time on during the course of a week. Okay, so, let's say you spend most of your time at work or school. After you get home, you most likely get onto a screen of some sort, your phone, laptop, PS4 – whatever, until you go to bed and start it all over again the next morning. You may spend time with your partner, friends, or kids. Maybe you work-out or have something else you like doing – reading, painting, photography? Now, think about how much time you're spending on each activity in terms of hours. Got it?

The next step involves reflecting on how much meaning what you're doing has for you. What do I mean by this? Think; is this important to you? Is it a priority? Does it bring you happiness? So, let's say you're spending most of your time at a job with little meaning to you, is there any way you can bring meaning to it or explore other opportunities? If you're spending the bulk of your day doing something that gives you little meaning, it's not serving you. Maybe you really value your family, but find you're too burnt out at night to do little else than veg out in front of a screen. How can you change that? Or, you have something that gives you tremendous meaning but devote little of your time doing it? You want to be fit and healthy, but never find the time or motivation? I know we all have "reasons" why our time/value balance is out of whack. But here is the awesome thing; we can bring meaning to all we do. We can slowly make changes to ensure that we spend time doing things and do things with people that bring us true happiness, value, and meaning.

Is the way you're spending your time to reflect on what is important to you and what has meaning and brings you happiness? You may see that you are spending the majority of your free-time watching television or on your computer and very little time with your family, friends, or loved ones; even though you know that spending time with family brings you true happiness. Are you making sure you devote time to your physical and spiritual wellbeing each day? How you invest your time has a direct impact on how you feel about yourself, others, and life. It is important that you begin to cultivate habits and routines which lend themselves to you spending time doing things that have meaning and bring happiness. Begin phasing out activities that create negative emotions or leave you listless.

In his book, Emotional Intelligence, Daniel Goleman writes that "each successive generation worldwide since the opening of the twentieth century has lived with a higher risk than their parents of suffering a major depression – not just sadness, but a paralyzing listlessness, dejection, self-pity, and an overwhelming hopelessness over the course of life." The overwhelming hopelessness, the nihilism, that Goleman describes results from our sense that we are unable to achieve true happiness and meaning in our lives.

With this hopelessness comes some of our most disturbing social problems, including substance abuse. It is easy to see why an unhappy person might turn to substances, if they provide a temporary escape from the reality of life.

There is a direct relationship on how increasing our happiness improves our quality of life and in turn, improves the positive impact we have on our communities as a whole.

We can see how this relationship impacts individuals and communities. When there is widespread unhappiness and a loss of connection with our self, others, and the Divine, mental un-wellness and mental illness increases because we aren't truly happy. And, guess what? Substance abuse rates rise! Through this lens, happiness is seen not as some fleeting emotion but as something important and vital to be pursued to increase the overall wellness of ourselves and the communities in which we live.

Setting Goals

Happiness grows less from the passive experience of desirable circumstances than from involvement in valued activities and progress toward one's goals.
– David Myers and Ed Diener

Goals are indispensable to a happy life – to be happy, we need to identify and pursue goals that feel good and are meaningful. Goals communicate to ourselves and to others the belief that we are capable of overcoming obstacles and accomplishing what we set out minds to. It says, "I believe in me!" A goal, an explicit commitment, focuses our attention on the target and helps us to find ways of getting there. Goals are self-fulfilling prophecies and when we commit to one, we demonstrate faith in ourselves and in our ability to achieve an envisioned future. We create our reality rather than react to it. As we reach our goals, we begin to feel empowered and shed the victim mentality we have been hiding under. When we see that we are in the driver's seat, we can determine our goals, our thoughts, and our actions. In this sense, although, the actual fulfillment of goals brings us happiness, the simple act of setting goals is actually equally important.

In this way, goals liberate us so that we can enjoy the here and now. The emphasis becomes not so much on attaining goals, but acknowledging and owning that we have the ability and desire to set goals and achieve them.

Goals are a means, not just an end. For long term happiness, we need to change the expectations we have of our goals. The work we do on the journey toward achieving our goals is incredibly valuable. We learn so much about ourselves. We develop strengths, self-esteem, confidence, and knowledge. Each step we take to attain our goals increases our wellbeing. It's a win-win situation. Okay, here's a very simplistic example. Take, for instance, someone who is trying to lose ten pounds. Losing the weight doesn't happen overnight; it may take months, but with each day a mindfulness of how to care for your body is developed. In this sense, it isn't the weight loss that is so important. It's the process of developing healthy, positive behaviours to achieve the desired end goal that ends up serving you in the long run. You are re-enforcing the idea that you are worthy of the daily effort needed to reach the goal and you have the capacity to achieve! The journey becomes the gift!

Self-Concordant Goals

Self-concordant goals are those we pursue out of deep personal conviction or passion. There is a huge difference between the meaning we get from extrinsic goals, external things; like wealth and social status, and the meaning we get from intrinsic goods, such as personal growth and a sense of connection with others.

It's great to have career goals and there is no shame in wanting material things. The trouble is when we believe that without those things, we are less worthy. You know the old cliché money can't buy happiness; well, on a deeper level, this is true. Of course, it's great to have abundance enough to live a healthy, content life. But if we aren't connected to our true Self, we still feel lack. That's why it's important to set intrinsic goals; goals that bring happiness to your mind, your heart, and your spirit self. Think of these as your true goals. When we follow our true wants and goals, we not only enjoy the journey, but we are also more happy. Without a clear and personally compelling sense of direction, it becomes easy to feel, as though, we are aimless meandering and we get pulled away from our real, authentic self. When we know where we are going and know what we truly want, it is much easier for us to stay on course, true to ourselves. We are more likely to listen to the voice coming from within.

Remember that whether or not you actually achieve your goals is not the most important factor for long-term happiness. The primary objective of goals is to liberate you to your true Self; enabling you to enjoy the present, the here, and now.

Action Plan

What do you need to do in the coming month, week, or day to support both your short and long term goals? In your calendar, put down the actual activities that you need to carry out in order to begin the journey. Sound simple? Well, it is! And guess what? The act of putting thought into reality, putting our intention out to the universe propels us to action.

When we do not set clear goals for ourselves, we are at the mercy of external forces, which rarely lead to self-concordant activities. The choice we face is between passively reacting to the world in which we live or actively creating our life.

Self-Esteem

Self-esteem is a way of thinking, feeling, and acting that shows you accept, respect, trust, and believe in yourself. When you accept yourself just as you are, you are able to live with both your personal strengths and weaknesses, without all of the negative self-talk. When you respect yourself, you acknowledge your own dignity and value as a unique human being. To believe in yourself means that you feel you deserve to have the good things in life. It also means that you have the confidence that you can fulfill your deepest personal needs, aspirations, and goals.

It's pretty incredible, really. We are self-contained units of infinite potential!

A fundamental truth about self-esteem is that it needs to come from within. When self-esteem is low, it creates a feeling of emptiness that you may try to fill – often compulsively – with something external that provides a temporary sense of satisfaction and fulfillment. We often look to fill our inner emptiness through bonding with something outside ourselves in a way that can become desperate, repetitive, or automatic. It moves beyond healthy into addiction. Think of it this way; addiction is an attachment or bonding to something, or someone outside yourself that you feel you need to provide a sense of inner satisfaction or relief. Unfortunately, this need often substitutes unhealthy behaviours or substances for healthy human relationships. When we're in this place, we substitute a temporary feeling of control or power for a more lasting sense of inner confidence and strength.

Building your self-esteem, a sense of self, is necessary to let go of the addiction. Growing in self-esteem means developing confidence and strength from within. When you can do this, you are still enjoying life fully and you no longer need something or someone outside yourself to make you feel worthy. The basis for your self-worth is internal. Because of this, it has the potential to be long lasting and stable.

There are many pathways to self-esteem. It is not something that develops overnight. It is built gradually – step by step, day by day, small goal to small goal.

Be kind to yourself during this time, you are worthy!

Your willingness and ability to take care of yourself is fundamental to your self-esteem. This applies to both your basic needs as a human and to your emotional and spiritual needs. Learning to meet your needs – to care for and nurture yourself – is the most fundamental and important thing you can do to build your self-esteem.

When I speak of basic human needs, I mean things like shelter, food, clothing, food, water, sleep, and basic hygiene care. When you finally get to a place where you're clean and sober, it's often frightening to think back to how far you let yourself go in terms of self-care. Even basic daily care is thrown out the window. When you're in this dark place, your spiritual and emotional life takes a back seat to addiction. You're in survival mode; doing what you need, just to get by, and sustain the addiction. Here's the kicker: while our spiritual life, happiness, and self-esteem can't pay the bills, without them, it's hard to get to a place where we have enough belief in ourselves to live a life of purpose and value – to envision a life worth living without substances.

So what do we need to live a fulfilled life beyond our basic human needs? Have a look at the following list. How many of these needs are being met in your life right now?

1. Physical safety and security
2. Financial security
3. Friendship
4. The attention of others
5. Being listened to
6. Guidance
7. Respect
8. Validation
9. Expressing and sharing your feelings
10. Sense of belonging
11. Nurturing
12. Physically touching and being touched
13. Intimacy
14. Sexual expression
15. Loyalty and trust
16. A sense of accomplishment
17. A sense of progress toward goals
18. Feeling competent or masterful in some area
19. Making a contribution
20. Fun and play
21. Sense of freedom and independence
22. Creativity
23. Spiritual awareness; connection with a Higher Power
24. Unconditional love

What do you notice when you look at the list? Do you feel many of your needs are being met? Do you notice any connections or patterns in certain areas? I want you to think of steps you can take in the next few weeks and months to better meet those needs that are going unmet. Even acknowledging we have needs that aren't being met can be uncomfortable. That's okay. We live in a world where we are raised to be so self-critical. It's really hard for us to acknowledge our wants and needs and that we deserve to have them met. Know it is okay to be uncomfortable. The whole point of the list is to recognize we have a wide variety of needs that we want to have met. Now, the challenge comes in thinking how you can begin to work toward one or two things on the list which are most important to you. Remember, start off small with attainable day to day goals that will and with time, reach an end objective.

Part of meeting our needs is to learn to truly love ourselves. If you were to encounter a small child who appeared scared, confused, or abandoned, you would likely do everything in your power to nurture and comfort him or her. Yet, how do you treat yourself when you feel insecure, scared, lonely, abandoned, or otherwise, needy? Too often we simply deny these feelings or we become self-critical, or we reject ourselves for having these feelings. We turn to substances to "forget" them. One of the most profound transformations you can make in cultivating greater self-esteem is to reframe feelings of insecurity and inadequacy as a sign that the inner you, your true Self, your inner child needs to be nurtured. You will heal yourself faster by acknowledging and nurturing these negative feelings rather than trying to avoid experiencing them and exploring their root cause. When we take this approach of denial and neglect, we miss out on the opportunity to take the power away from these negative emotions and their crippling effect they have had on us; preventing us from meeting our true needs.

The next time you feel frightened, insecure, inadequate, vulnerable, angry, frustrated, and fed up, try asking yourself "What is the need behind this feeling?"

Then, take the time to give this need the attention, caring, and nurturing you lack. Learn to re-perceive your negative feelings and emotions as a call to attention to your unmet needs.

The following is a beautiful visualization to help you develop a closer relationship with the inner you, the child in you. Take a moment to get comfortable in a quiet place, wherever you won't be interrupted for the next few minutes while you read the following:

Imagine sitting down in a rocking chair and getting very comfortable. Feel yourself rocking easily back and forth. As you continue rocking, you find yourself starting to drift...drifting more and more. Rocking back and forth, you find yourself gently drifting back into time. Rocking gently and drifting...slowly drifting back into time. Year by year, you imagine yourself getting younger and younger. The years are going by...gently drifting, feeling younger and younger. Slowly, your thoughts drift back to a time when you were very young. You're imaging now that you can see the little child you were a long time ago. What do you look like? What are you wearing? How old are you? Can you see where you are? Indoors or outdoors? Can you see what you're doing? You can see your face and if you look carefully, you can see the expression in your eyes. Can you tell how this little child is feeling right now? As you look at this little person, can you recall anything that was missing in your life? Is there anything that kept you from being fully happy? If there was anyone or anything that got in the way of this little girl being completely happy and carefree, perhaps, you can imagine seeing that person or situation. If no one is there yet, perhaps, you can imagine your dad or your mom or whomever you would like standing in front of you right now. What do you feel toward your dad, mom, or whomever is standing in front of you right now? Is there anything that your child would like to say to that person right now? If so, it's okay to go ahead and say it right now... you can go ahead and say it. You are safe here.

If your little child is feeling scared or confused about saying anything, imagine that your present-day, adult self enters the scene right now and goes up, and stands next to your little child. Now, when you're ready, imagine you're standing next to your little child, speaking up on your little child's behalf to whomever is there. Your adult self can say whatever you want. Tell your parent – or whoever is there – whatever you need to say...whatever it was that never got expressed. When you speak up, speak loud and clear so you can be sure that whoever is there, really hears you. Does the person you're facing have any response? Listen to see if they have a response. If so, you can respond to what they say. If not, you can just finish what you need to say. When you're finished speaking, you can ask whoever is there to either go away or leave you alone or to go away for a while until you're ready to talk again, or else ask them to stay. You're going to accept them as they are and give them a hug.

Now go back and see your present-day, adult self standing next to your child self. If you are willing, pick that little child up in your arms this very second and love them. Wrap your arms around them and tell them that it's okay. Tell them that you know how they feel. Tell them that you understand. You're here and you're going to help them, and you love them very, very much.

If you could give a colour to the love you feel, what colour comes to mind?

Surround your little child with a light of that colour and let them feel the peace of being in your arms. Tell them that you think they're incredible, that you love the way they talk, the way they walk, laugh...does everything. Tell them that you care and that you are precious.

And now, take a moment to ground yourself before continuing.

Intention

Our intent governs how we think, feel, and behave. Our intent is a powerful and creative force. It's the essence of free will. Your intent is your deepest desire, your primary motive or goal, your highest priority in any given moment. Having said that, there are really only two primary intents:

To learn about loving yourself and others, even in the face of fear and pain, or to protect yourself from fear and pain with addictive, controlling behaviour, and trying to avoid responsibility for your feelings and actions.

When your intent is to learn to love, you are willing to face your fears and experience your painful feelings in order to compassionately nurture them. The deeper purpose here is to become a more loving human being, starting with yourself. When you open yourself to learning about your own fear and beliefs and about what brings you joy, you move toward love. When the intent is to learn, learning about love becomes more important than protecting against fear. When your intent is to learn to love, your deepest desire is to find your safety, peace, lovability, and worth, through an internal connection with the unconditional love that is available on the spiritual level.

When your intent is to protect yourself from fear and pain, and avoid owning your feelings, your deepest desire is to find your safety, peace, lovability, and worth, through externals, like attention, approval, sex, substances, things, and activities. When our intention is to avoid our feelings, we look to others to bring us happiness. In this sense, because we look to others to escape our negative emotions or to make us happy, we believe that others are responsible for how we feel, we try to control others so they act in ways that will make us feel good about ourselves and allow us to avoid working through our negative emotions.

In every moment, each one of us chooses our intent; either to attempt to feel externally safe by controlling others and our own feelings, or to create inner safety by learning about loving ourselves and others. While the choices that others make may influence you, no one but you has control over your intent. In each moment, you choose what is most important to you and in each moment, you have an opportunity to change your mind and heart.

The intent to protect ourselves from pain and hurt closes the heart in an attempt to avoid feelings of loneliness, heartache, heartbreak, grief, sorrow, anger and helplessness over others. But, closing the heart to protect against these painful feelings leaves you feeling alone inside. To avoid and prevent further pain and hurt, we often think we can simply control our way out of it. You may even try to have control over getting love with criticism, blame, silence, or by giving in to others. You may avoid pain by retreating inward, resisting help, numbing out with food, drugs, alcohol, gambling, and screens. The more you try to have control over getting love and avoiding pain, the worse you feel and the more you do it to try to feel better. It's a vicious cycle.

In this way, the essence of self-esteem is compassion for yourself. When you have compassion for yourself, you understand and accept yourself. If you make a mistake, you forgive yourself. When you live to feel compassion for yourself, you begin exposing your sense of worth. You literally uncover the light within, casting light on the darkness.

Compassion

Compassion isn't something you either have or don't have. You have to actively work to cultivate compassion; it's not an unchanging trait. Most people think of compassion as a positive character trait, like honesty or loyalty; you either have it or you don't. If you have compassion, you show it by being kind, sympathetic, and helpful to yourself and others.

But here's the thing; you can develop compassion, if you lack it or increase it, if you already have it. Compassion is not only something you feel for others. It should also inspire you to be kind, sympathetic, and helpful to one's self.

There are three basic ways to cultivate compassion: understanding, acceptance, and forgiveness.

Understanding

An attempt to understand is the first step toward a compassionate relationship with yourself and others. Understanding something important about yourself or a loved one can totally change your feelings and attitudes.

Not all understanding comes easily. Sometimes, it comes as the result of a plodding, sustained effort to figure things out. It may come as the result of a negative event or circumstance.

Understanding the nature of the problem doesn't mean that you also have the solution. It simply means that you have a sense of how things have come to be and how you have come to be the person that you are.

Acceptance

Acceptance is perhaps the most difficult aspect of compassion. Acceptance is an acknowledgement of the situation as it is, of the facts, with all value judgments suspended. You neither approve nor disapprove; you simply accept. Sounds easy, but it is so hard to do. But just because it's hard, doesn't mean it isn't a practice well worth developing. Sometimes we simply need to understand how a situation has developed, acknowledge it, and that's enough, nothing more is needed.

Forgiveness

Forgiveness flows out of understanding and accepting. It means letting go of the past, reaffirming your self-worth in the present, and moving toward a positive future. When you forgive yourself for your addictions, you're not denying your past. You are moving away from a place that doesn't serve you to a place that does. You remember to move forward to live a peaceful today and have hope for tomorrow. True forgiveness of yourself and others means the account is balanced. The person who harmed or wronged you no longer owes you anything. And equally important, you no longer need to punish yourself for your wrongs.

You face the future with a fresh slate and a new beginning.

It is essential that we have compassion toward others as well as ourselves. In this moment, it may be easier for you to understand, accept, and forgive others than to forgive yourself. You will never be able to move forward until you understand that you are not your addictions. Accept where you were, without judgment and forgive yourself. Forgiveness in this sense is possible not through denial, but through love.

You may find you have compassion for others but struggle to let go of the hurt or disappointments in yourself. That's okay. If loving yourself seems really challenging, start with feeling compassion for others. Begin to understand, accept, and forgive others, first. It will bring light to your own greatness.

Getting Started

For four consecutive weeks, you will be asked to devote time each day to yoga, meditation, physical activity, and reflection. Every week will have a focus. On at least six days of each week, you will practice yoga and spend some time sitting in meditation.

You will also spend time integrating what you notice about yourself and your daily life. This integration is very important. It gives you the opportunity to get in touch with both your physical and spiritual self, something which has been missing in your life. To effectively take control of your health and wellness, you need to become more aware of what is happening in your life and what needs to change in your day-to-day routine.

How important is it to you to change your life? If it's important, then it's worth making the commitment to put aside the time for you to focus on wellness, through this work. But you have to decide that. I don't say this from some "tough love" kind of approach to recovery. I say this because we both know it's the truth. No matter how much support and encouragement you're given, it will never work unless you truly want wellness for yourself. Believe me, I do not believe in tough love. I think the whole notion is counter intuitive, truly. Tough has no place in the business of love. Let's call tough love what it really is; self-preservation and protection, a fear of others being hurt by our addiction or alcoholism.

One suggestion I have to help you keep your commitment is to take it one day at a time. As you look at your calendar for tomorrow, decide when you'll take the time to make this a priority in your day, above everything else you do. This will require some thought and effort. There are all kinds of good reasons we come up with for putting other things in front of ourselves. Don't compromise. Each day, schedule your commitment for the following day. You can give yourself a day off after you've completed six days in one week. But, if you want to practice on all seven days to keep a routine going, that's amazing, too!

It's a great idea to get the support of your friends and family. Let them know what you are doing and why you are doing it, and ask for their encouragement. Ultimately, your success will be dependent on your own willingness to make this program a priority for four weeks and to make changes in your life that promote wellness and let you take control of your body, and experience more joy.

Where Will You Find the Time?

Now that you are ready commit time to you, you're probably wondering, "How am I ever going to do this?" My thought is that if this is really important to you, you'll create the time. In my life with children, a partner, job, our home, and other responsibilities, the day seems to get very busy after 8 a.m. My mind also gets busy and it's easy for me to make excuses that I have more urgent things to do other than spend time on my physical and spiritual wellbeing. So, if I'm going to take time for myself, it usually has to be early in the morning or late in the evening.

You have to decide when you can find the time. You may find it helpful to do this practice at the same time and in the same place every day. The important thing is to just do it. If you are reading this, it is because you are ready to do what is required to make yourself a priority, to value, and love yourself enough to give you the time needed to nurture you to make you feel better and cultivate more joy in your life. And, realistically, you used to spend a lot of time feeding your addiction and alcoholism. You now have all of that time to devote to things that will serve you positively.

As you begin to notice the positive changes that come to you from this program, the temptation to drop it and go back to old ways can be very strong. This is because change doesn't happen overnight. One change invites more changes and in many areas in life. Think of your own life; you didn't get to this place overnight, it developed over time. The same is true of recovery. Be patient. This is not an overnight solution. Be kind to yourself and love yourself enough to commit to a healthy life – mind, body, and spirit.

Some of the things you will be doing along with your exercise program are drinking and eating mindfully, walking, performing self-care exercises, performing small acts of kindness for others and yourself, journaling, and learning more about yourself. Each week will have a focused theme and each day of that week will contain exercises and tasks.

My intention is help you develop a mindful approach to your daily life. Because of this, how you do things is just as important as what you are doing. Make sense? You will be asked to do things mindfully. This means really noticing what happens moment to moment, while you work the program. You will soon see this practice carry over into the rest of your daily activities. When you are clear about the choices you are making, then you can adapt and make different choices, which will positively impact your health and wellness. You are now in a place blessed with choice. You are clean, you are present, and you are able to choose things to strengthen and empower your journey. That's an incredible gift! You can choose things that serve you! You are not controlled by a substance or by others. You have the power of choice. Choose you! You are worthy!

Why All of These Push-Ups?

Okay, so, first, it is yoga and now, its push-ups, crunches and drinking lots of water each day. You're probably wondering what any of this has to do with the journey you are on. I knew that it would be important to explain why I am including this as part of the work we are doing. I know that this may seem simplistic and boring, but there is a method to my madness. These basic exercises are ones that most of us have done at some point in our lives. We may have always dreaded them in phys-ed class, but we know what they are.

And guess what? We can all do them! They may not be pretty. We may not do many of them, we may even hate them – we may have struggled and moaned, and groaned, but that is going to change.

The water will keep you hydrated and flush out toxins.

It is my intention to make this program accessible and the goals attainable for everyone. That means there are no excuses! There is no need to go to a gym or purchase any equipment, in order to do what is being asked of you. Know that everyone finds push-ups and crunches challenging, but here is the beauty; over time, with consistent effort, you will see that they begin to become easier. You will begin to struggle less and perhaps, do more. You will see yourself become stronger. There will be measurable changes. You will see the direct correlation between effort and results. And, here is the other incredible thing; the first time you do even just few push-ups or crunches, you will come away with a sense of accomplishment. A seed will be planted. As you continue to persevere with yoga and the program, you will begin to become aware that you have the capacity to do! You can do it. Know that you are becoming stronger, more determined. Through the connection with your physical self, you will begin to develop a deep, lasting relationship with the spiritual self. Your sense of self-worth and determination will grow and strengthen. With each day, you will cultivate feelings of value; feelings in the positive realm, not the negative. You will begin to feel worthy of self-care and self-love. In acknowledging and caring for the physical self, you are laying the foundation on which your loving, your inner self can flourish.

Oh yeah, for fun, take the bliss test at the back of the book and tuck it away until the end of the program!

Please visit carrieschell.com There you can download the yoga sequence using the code MBSYOGA. You can also download the guided meditations to start you on your journey. Use the code MBSMEDITATION.

Before We Begin...

Let the light in me, light and honour the light in you...
Namaste.

Week One

Week One

Here is your first week's schedule. I have marked the start of the program as Sunday for simplicity; a fresh start, but that's just me. Feel free to start on whatever day you like.

The theme for this first week is befriending your body.

Your body is a key player in your success with this program. It is through your body that you will learn the most and through your body that you will change everything in your life that needs to change. This first week will guide you to reconnect with your physical self and explore where your body is at. It will be the foundation to developing a loving relationship with yourself and discovering your sense of self and self-worth.

The first question you need to ask yourself is, "What kind of relationship do I have with my body?" And before you jump with a negative response, take time to really investigate this. If you do have negative thoughts about your body, how did this happen? At what point in your life did you start being negative about you? At what point in your life did you give yourself permission to be out of shape and harm your body with lack of exercise and poor eating? We all struggle with body issues. I can tell you that this is a strong barrier for me. I struggle to like my body and am working to accept and love how I look. Over the next four weeks of our work together, and I emphasize together, we will learn from each other. Our goal is to feel better, to be in control and on the path to a fit and healthy life physically, emotionally, and spiritually.

Putting Intent into Action

This and every other week of the program, as you begin to become more aware of yourself and how you are showing up in your life, you will have the opportunity to try out new ideas that come to you during your practice – particularly in the reflective exercises of journaling and meditation. See if you can find ways to put new awareness to work for you in your daily life. It may be as simple as deciding you want to smile more or share a kind word to a loved one, or give your child or partner a hug. Simple things, such as these, may not look like life changing acts, but if you repeat them daily and practice them with conscious awareness, they will go a long way in supporting you, as you turn your stress into bliss.

SUNDAY

Before you get out of bed, before your feet hit the floor, simply say, "Thank you. I am blessed. I am grateful."

Do this every morning when you awake.

You may simply be saying this and initially, it may have little meaning and it may ring hollow, but give it time. Each day you are substance free, these simple phrases will mean more and more to you. You are here, against the odds. Thank you for being here! I am blessed and full of gratitude to be part of your journey.

Five Minutes

Begin your day with sitting quietly for five minutes. Do not focus on your day and the tasks at hand. Simply sit and breathe.

Thirty Minutes

Devote twenty minutes to any cardio activity that you choose. Put in a DVD, attend a class, or go for a power walk. I want you to feel your breathing intensify, to a point where it is getting challenging to speak while doing your cardio. This is a great gauge; that you are in your target cardio heart rate zone.

> 20 push-ups; these can be wall push-ups, knee push-ups, or plank push-ups as demonstrated in class. Key pointers; keep the back straight, not arched. Abdominals engaged and neck in neutral spine position.
> 20 crunches: these are great for the abdominals and core. You may have your hands on the ground or active in the exercise as well.

20 squats: key for your quads, core, and butt. Feet shoulder width apart, back straight, and core engaged. Enjoy!

Practice yoga with me...pop in the DVD and enjoy a guided meditation.

Drink eight glasses of water today. Water? Yuk! Try it, you'll like it! The water will help cleanse your system and flush your liver, removing toxins from your body. Do it, your body will love you.

Journaling

You will be journaling daily. I want you to record everything you eat for the next week. Why do I want you to do this? Well, for many of us, with or without weight issues, eating mindfully has not been a priority. Forget priority, eating mindfully hasn't been on the radar. By actually writing down what you eat, you draw your attention to what you are putting into your body. You are cultivating awareness of what you eat. Through awareness, you can begin to make conscious choices, which will support a healthy you. So, no cheating here! It is important for you to get a handle on what you eat, when you eat, how much you are eating, and even, why you eat. I also want you to record how the exercises felt. I would like you to write down one positive thing that you like about yourself and one positive thing about the day ahead of you.

Perform one small act to support your intention of befriending your body, like put the chocolate bar down! This can be something as simple as not criticizing yourself today or maybe, you'll make an effort to smile more. Maybe you'll call a friend you've been thinking about. One small act of kindness that signals you are worthy.

Schedule something special for you for Wednesday night – a walk, a bubble bath, a yummy dinner, or a movie out!

Today's thought...

If you don't accept yourself, you won't life fully and if you don't live fully, you'll need to get full some other way.

Accepting who you are, body and soul, does not guarantee that you will be perfect. It does, however, put you in the ideal position for becoming truly happy and healthy, developing habits to last a lifetime. If you don't accept yourself, you won't live fully and, if you don't live fully, you'll need to get full some other way and unfortunately, it's usually with things that don't support you.

Word for today: DENIAL (Don't Even Notice I'm Living)

Denial is a defense mechanism. It protects us from the truth; especially, when the truth is painful. We do not want to see reality because of what it ultimately means. For us, the truth is that we are not able to drink or use other drugs, we are not who we thought we were. Our self-esteem cannot face this harsh reality, so we alter our reality. We pretend to be something we are not. We cannot accept reality's limitations. Denial needs to be penetrated or shattered before we can truly admit that we are totally powerless over alcohol and other drugs.

– Allen Berger, *12 Stupid Things That Mess Up Recovery.*

Affirmation: I am now willing to acknowledge the truth of my addiction.

Exercise: Reveal to yourself how often you have lied, both to yourself and others, in order to cover your addiction. Remember that this is for your eyes only and it is of vital importance that you are on this journey with honesty.

_____

_____

_____

_____

_____

_____

_____

_____

_____

_____

_____

_____

_____

_____

_____

_____

_____

MONDAY

Five Minutes

Begin your day with sitting quietly for five minutes. Do not focus on your day and the tasks at hand. Simply sit and breathe.

Thirty Minutes

Devote twenty minutes to any cardio activity that you choose. Put in a DVD, attend a class, or go for a power walk. I want you to feel your breathing intensify to a point where it is getting challenging to speak while doing your cardio. This is a great gauge that you are in your target cardio heart rate zone.

20 push-ups: these can be wall push-ups, knee push-ups, or plank push-ups as demonstrated in class. Key pointers: keep the back straight, not arched. Abdominals engaged and neck in neutral spine position.

20 crunches: these are great for the abdominals and core. You may have your hands on the ground or active in the exercise as well.

20 squats: key for your quads, core, and butt. Feet shoulder width apart, back straight, and core engaged. Enjoy!

Practice yoga with me. Pop in the DVD and enjoy a guided meditation!

Drink eight glasses of water today.

Remember, your body will love it!

Journaling

You will be journaling daily. I want you to record everything you eat for the next week. No cheating here! This is important for you to get a handle on what you eat, when you eat, how much you are eating, and perhaps, why you eat. I also want you to record how the exercises felt. I would like you to write down one positive thing that you like about yourself and one positive thing about the day ahead of you.

Perform one small act to support your intention of befriending your body. Find the time to work-out.

Today's thought…

You can eat better and still be yourself.

Why all the food talk? Believe it or not, there is a connection between what you eat and how you feel about yourself. The more you become aware of your worthiness, of how great you are, the more likely you are to begin to eat healthy. They go hand in hand. That's why we're spending some time developing a positive attitude toward food and eating. You can adopt better habits only if you honour who you are. There is a healthy way of eating that is natural and realistic for you. The point is to know yourself, respect yourself, and make appropriate choices based on who you are and how you live. When you make the changes that will nurture change for your body and your life, they have to be the ones that work for you and that honour who you are. It may take some adjustments and there may be some painful bumps along the way, but you are worth the effort. The point is to have a healthier lifestyle, not to live a life full of resentments due to newly adopted changes.

Ask Yourself:

What does reasonable eating look like to me?

How much time do I want to spend preparing food?

What challenges to improve the way I eat, does my job present?

Will my spouse or family be a help or hindrance to my making these changes?

Am I feeding children throughout the day?

Do I have a health condition that requires me to eat in a certain way?

These are all things to consider on the road to healthy eating.

As you are painfully aware, what we put into our bodies has an incredible impact on all aspects of our lives. The same is true with food. It can either support us or harm us.

Word for today: FEAR (False Experiences Appearing Real)

The dark giants of fear and ignorance are closely allied. For instance; it's within no one's power to slay fear, because fear exists only as a shadow of the unknown and shadows can't be slain. But it is within our power to challenge and conquer what is unknown, since nothing can prevent us from learning.

— Guy Finley, *The Secret of Letting Go*

Affirmation: I am now willing to be courageous.

Exercise: Reveal to yourself the underlying fears of letting go of your addiction. For example; are you frightened of the withdrawals, of your real feelings without the buffer of a substance, or perhaps, you fear losing the courage you feel your substance gives you?

_____

_____

_____

_____

_____

_____

_____

_____

_____

_____

_____

_____

_____

_____

_____

TUESDAY

Five Minutes

Begin your day with sitting quietly for five minutes. Do not focus on your day and the tasks at hand. Simply sit and breathe.

Thirty Minutes

Devote twenty minutes to any cardio activity that you choose. Put in a DVD, attend a class, or go for a power walk. I want you to feel your breathing intensify to a point where it is getting challenging to speak while doing your cardio. This is a great gauge that you are in your target cardio heart rate zone.

20 push-ups: these can be wall push-ups, knee push-ups, or plank push-ups as demonstrated in class. Key pointers: keep the back straight, not arched. Abdominals engaged and neck in neutral spine position.

20 ins and outs: these are great for the abdominals and core. You may have your hands on the ground or active in the exercise as well.

20 squats: key for your quads, core, and butt. Feet shoulder width apart, back straight, and core engaged. Enjoy!

Drink eight glasses of water today.

Practice yoga with me. Pop in the DVD!

Enjoy a guided meditation.

Journaling

You will be journaling daily. I want you to record everything you eat for the next week. No cheating here! This is important for you to get a handle on what you eat, when you eat, how much you are eating, and perhaps, why you eat. I also want you to record how the exercises felt. I would like you to write down one positive thing that you like about yourself and one positive thing about the day ahead of you.

Perform one small act to support your intention of befriending your body. Tell yourself "I want to be healthy" fifty times today.

How are your plans coming for doing something special and healthy for you, tomorrow night? Give it some thought. Small acts of kindness toward yourself are so important.

Today's thought...

Give up the notion of blowing it!

This one simple phrase unknowingly signals, both, defeat on our path to wellness and permission to continue in unhealthy behaviours all at once, really! Think of it in terms of dieting. The simple sentence "I blew it" may be responsible for more weight gained than all of the french fries at McDonalds. It goes like this, "It's Friday. I ate really well all week. But then, I cheated and ate a cookie (chips, chocolate bar, whatever). I blew it. I'll start fresh Monday. So, now, I have to eat for three days and be really miserable!" Okay, so, you had a cookie. Fine. I hope it tasted good. I hope you left some in the bag for someone else. Either way, it's done. Get your brain out of your stomach and go do something interesting. Give yourself permission to do it differently.

The "blowing it" concept is a setup. It's a mind game we play to give ourselves permission to lapse for a fix. If you blow it, you don't have to throw in the towel thinking sobriety is forever out of reach.

Instead, don't blow it! Easier said than done, I know. But there are two ways you can do this. One is to keep your expectations realistic, so you will reach them. Back to our food analogy. For example: aspiring to each three reasonable meals today and get your exercise in, is realistic. Setting your sights on running ten km daily and eating only skinless chicken and lettuce leaves for the next four weeks, isn't. So, be kind to yourself in these early days and do not place yourself in situations that will trigger use and set you up for failure. Out of sight, out of mind...slowly and gradually. Eventually, you will get to a place where you are not thinking and craving continually. You will begin to have experiences that do not require alcohol or drugs to be enjoyable, or of perceived value.

The other way to stop blowing it is to disallow the concept itself. Let's say you slept in and couldn't get your exercise in for today. Did you blow it? No! Unless you decide to give yourself permission to eat junk food only and to never exercise again, then you have "blown it." So, you missed your work out or had that piece of cake. Give yourself a different response: "Yeah, you didn't work out (or I ate the cake). Sometimes, that will happen. Let it go!" That single change will alter the negative pattern.

The key is to acknowledge the problem and get right back at it! Don't continue to over eat for the rest of the day, or until Monday, the famous diet start date! You had a slip. Do not give yourself permission to derail completely. Commit to bettering yourself in that moment. Tell yourself I had a slipup, but you know what? I love myself enough to move on, move forward, and continue my wellness journey. Call a friend. Call a sponsor. Go to a meeting. Go to Church. Go for a walk or a hike. Get out in nature. Do whatever you need to do to reconnect with your inner-self that wants a substance free life. Continue with the program this very moment. And most importantly, forgive yourself.

Love yourself.

Word for today: ANXIETY

Start suspecting that those anxious thoughts and feelings you catch trying to sell you an umbrella are not there to shelter you from some approaching storm...but, that their sole purpose is to lure you into one.

– Guy Finley, The Secret Way of Wonder

Affirmation: I am now willing to have a quiet mind, an open heart, and relaxed body.

Exercise: Reveal to yourself how you have used your addiction to release or suppress anxious thoughts and feelings. Be honest with how your substance abuse has impacted your health, physically, mentally, and emotionally.

_____

_____

_____

_____

_____

_____

_____

_____

_____

_____

_____

_____

_____

_____

_____

_____

WEDNESDAY

Five Minutes

Begin your day with sitting quietly for five minutes. Do not focus on your day and the tasks at hand. Simply sit and breathe.

Thirty Minutes

Devote twenty minutes to any cardio activity that you choose. Put in a DVD, attend a class, or go for a power walk. I want you to feel your breathing intensify to a point where it is getting challenging to speak while doing your cardio. This is a great gauge that you are in your target cardio heart rate zone.

20 push-ups: these can be wall push-ups, knee push-ups, or plank push-ups, as demonstrated in class. Key pointers: keep the back straight, not arched. Abdominals engaged and neck in neutral spine position.

20 ins and outs: these are great for the abdominals and core. You may have your hands on the ground or active in the exercise as well.

20 squats: key for your quads, core, and butt. Feet shoulder width apart, back straight, and core engaged. Enjoy!

Practice yoga with me. Pop in the DVD and enjoy a guided meditation!

Drink eight glasses of water today.

Journaling

You will be journaling daily. I want you to record everything you eat for the next week. No cheating here! This is important for you to get a handle on what you eat, when you eat, how much you are eating, and perhaps, why you eat. I also want you to record how the exercises felt. I would like you to write down one positive thing that you like about yourself and one positive thing about the day ahead of you.

Perform one small act to support your intention of befriending your body. Put a post-it note on the fridge, "I want to be healthy. I am worth it, to not eat junk."

Enjoy the bubble bath!

Today's thought...

As a rule, eat three meals a day.

The act of having to eat three times daily serves us on many levels. In order to eat three times daily, we need to put thought and energy into what we are going to eat. You're actually going to have to be mindful throughout your day in how you are going to nurture your body. You'll be mindfully caring for yourself three times daily and that's huge! Not only will you be substance-free, you'll be filling your body with nutritious meals three times a day. Oh yeah, the meals are going to be healthy. No junk. No fast food. No refined sugars. No pop. Just whole, real foods! What? You may even find the planning and cooking of meals a welcomed addition to your day. If you're not in the position to cook or the thought of cooking makes you want to vomit, choose restaurants that serve "real," whole foods. No fast foods, seriously! Remember that packaged, low-fat, low calorie, supposedly, good for us foods are loaded with sugars and are so unhealthy. So, avoid them. Our brains react to refined sugars the same way it does to many drugs, especially cocaine. Four grams of sugar is equal to one teaspoon. So, that can of coke you love with 36 grams of sugar, that's nine teaspoons! My intention is supporting your journey to a substance-free, stronger, healthier you.

We are a breakfast, lunch, and dinner society. So, the idea of three meals a day fits. This doesn't mean that there can never be an exception; afternoon coffee with a friend or popcorn at the movies but as a rule, try to stick with eating three, reasonably sized meals per day. As we continue in the program, we will be modifying this notion as we gain more control over our eating habits and work towards kick starting our metabolism.

If you are able to stick to the three meals a day plan, there will be several hours during your day in which you will have nothing in your mouth. This is good. This is when you learn to focus on your inner life and your outer world.

Eating three meals a day is, both, a discipline and a gift. In the beginning, it might take all the fortitude you've got to get from one meal to the next, without picking up something to eat. Call on your inner resources, understanding friends, or pick up a book, anything to inspire and encourage you. Learn the difference between what feels like hunger and when you think you're hungry, because you are used to eating often. Don't skip meals, either. You want to establish a nice, comfortable rhythm.

One more thing; should your food get out of hand, you ate something really crappy or maybe you ate far too much or even had a down and out binge, it's all good. Just regroup. The temptation is to say, "I overate yesterday so today I won't eat at all," or "I'll skip breakfast and lunch and just have a light dinner." Don't. Get back to the three meals a day plan, as soon as you realize what happened. You don't have to eat a lot, but go through the motions of the routine. Have a meal, or part of one. Reinforce the act of positive behaviours; both, when things are going well and when things temporarily fall apart.

Word for today: SHAME

Shame is an isolating feeling. We keep it hidden. Yet, the more we isolate, hide it behind the masks that once served us, the bigger it grows and the lonelier we feel. The more shame we feel, the more fear we feel. The greater the shame, the greater the fear of being alone! It's a crazy cycle. We may even act out in anger or turn it inward in the form of depression. When we act out of fear and hurt others, we feel shame and begin the cycle all over again. It is important not to re-shame ourselves in the process of our recovery. The wounded child inside us doesn't need more injury. We need to start turning down the volume on those ghosts form the past. We need to be aware of any shaming from those who are currently in our lives, then take the hand of the wounded child inside us and lead her or him away. Above all, we need to begin to be aware when we are shaming ourselves.

— Jane Middleton-Moz, *Shame and Guilt*

Affirmation: I release the past and I am grateful for the lessons learned.

Exercise: Explain why you are so tired of feeling guilty.

_____

_____

_____

_____

_____

_____

_____

_____

_____

_____

_____

_____

_____

_____

_____

THURSDAY

Five Minutes

Begin your day with sitting quietly for five minutes. Do not focus on your day and the tasks at hand. Simply sit and breathe.

Thirty Minutes

Devote twenty minutes to any cardio activity that you choose. Put in a DVD, attend a class, or go for a power walk. I want you to feel your breathing intensify to a point where it is getting challenging to speak while doing your cardio. This is a great gauge; that you are in your target cardio heart rate zone.

20 push-ups; these can be wall push-ups, knee push-ups, or plank push-ups, as demonstrated in class. Key pointers: keep the back straight, not arched. Abdominals engaged and neck in neutral spine position.

20 ins and outs; these are great for the abdominals and core. You may have your hands on the ground or active in the exercise as well.

20 squats; key for your quads, core, and butt. Feet shoulder width apart, back straight, and core engaged. Enjoy!

Meet you on the yoga mat. Pop in the DVD and enjoy a guided meditation!

Drink eight glasses of water today.

Journaling

You will be journaling daily. I want you to record everything you eat for the next week. No cheating here! This is important for you to get a handle on what you eat, when you eat, how much you are eating, and perhaps, why you eat. I also want you to record how the exercises felt. I would like you to write down one positive thing that you like about yourself and one positive thing about the day ahead of you.

Perform one small act to support your intention of befriending your body. Buy a great piece of fruit for a snack.

Today's thought…

Set your intention for the day.

Before you get out of bed each morning, set your intention for the day. I know it sounds cliché, but give it a shot. At first, it is going to seem forced and, it will be. That doesn't matter. The act of setting a positive intention for your day; forced or not, will have a direct impact on you. Your intention can be simple, but make sure it is positive. You will begin to experience that beginning your day with positive intentions will actually set you up to have a good day. Remember, you create your thoughts and your thoughts create your reality. You have the power and choice to make your thoughts positive or negative. Your thoughts become your actions, which, in turn, become your reality. This is a huge concept and it can be; both, scary and liberating. Keep your heart and mind focused on positivity and gratitude, and you will be blown away with the changes you experience in life. Promise!

Word for today: ANGER.

Underneath your anger, your need to control, your need to blame your impatience, and your intolerance of others' weaknesses, is a great deal of pain. In fact, pain often causes you to become angry in the first place. If you find that you are angry most of the time and that your anger seems to linger on too long, take a peek underneath to see if there is pain that you have been voiding. If you don't expose your pain, you will never have a chance to heal. Instead, it will fester and worsen, causing you to become more bitter, defensive, angry, every day.

Affirmation: I choose peace.

Exercise: Did you grow up in an angry family? If not, describe what makes you angry and how you express anger. For example; yelling, silent treatment, or physical violence.

_____

_____

_____

_____

_____

_____

_____

_____

_____

_____

_____

_____

_____

_____

_____

_____

_____

FRIDAY

Five Minutes

Begin your day with sitting quietly for five minutes. Do not focus on your day and the tasks at hand. Simply sit and breathe.

Thirty Minutes

Devote twenty minutes to any cardio activity that you choose. Put in a DVD, attend a class, or go for a power walk. I want you to feel your breathing intensify to a point where it is getting challenging to speak while doing your cardio. This is a great gauge; that you are in your target cardio heart rate zone.

20 push-ups: these can be wall push-ups, knee push-ups, or plank push-ups, as demonstrated in class. Key pointers: keep the back straight, not arched. Abdominals engaged and neck in neutral spine position.

20 ins and outs: these are great for the abdominals and core. You may have your hands on the ground or active in the exercise as well.

20 squats: key for your quads, core, and butt. Feet shoulder width apart, back straight, and core engaged. Enjoy!

Let's do yoga together! Pop in the DVD and enjoy a guided meditation!

Drink eight glasses of water today.

Journaling

You will be journaling daily. I want you to record everything you eat for the next week. No cheating here! This is important for you to get a handle on what you eat, when you eat, how much you are eating, and perhaps, why you eat. I also want you to record how the exercises felt. I would like you to write down one positive thing that you like about yourself and one positive thing about the day ahead of you.

Perform one small act to support your intention of befriending your body (buy a great piece of fruit for a snack).

Today's thought...

Alter your definition of success.

Success is not something you acquire down the road. It can be precisely where you are on the journey, right now, today. Start to interpret success from a loving, more serving place. Success is every day you pay attention to your inner life, eat reasonably, respect your body, and treat yourself and others, well. Begin to recognize that success is found in your inner life. Once you begin to shift your success or sense of worthiness from externals and things to your inner life and relationships, you experience success in your everyday life.

Take a moment and ask yourself:

- Have I been kind to me today?
- Is how I am spending my time a reflection of what I value?
- Have I expressed gratitude to those I love?
- Am I mindful to stay in the positive?
- Have I taken care of my physical wellbeing today?
- And, this is the big one; am I acting from a source of fear or love?

Early on, having fear is normal. We live in a world that cultivates fears and struggles to believe in the higher power of love. Don't be afraid of being afraid. A bit of trepidation can even be a good thing – the way stage fright can lead to a better performance. But, fear can only serve us, if it propels us to move away from thinking and acting out of fear to a place where we are living from a source of love. Release your fears in your journal. Connect to your Higher Power through meditation, prayer, or spend some more time in nature.

The idea is to start living fully and being a success in your own eyes, sooner rather than later. You're succeeding in every moment, day by day. Remember that. You are entering a bright new world, where you will find more opportunities for fulfillment and joy. Expect this. Accept this as you are actively changing the state of your mind, body, and spirit.

Word for today: COMMUNICATION

Relationships are not optional. They are a necessity. As humans, we have an innate need to bond. If you cannot bond with others, you will bond with other things to try to meet that need; substances, shopping, food, sex, gambling, Facebook, whatever.

This is why you have to reach out to others. Being able to communicate with others is essential to building meaningful relationships and creating bonds with others.

The benefits of relationships are infinite and are key to our:

- Humanness
- Psychological health
- Personal identity
- Social, cognitive, and moral development
- Coping with stress and adversity
- Meaning to and quality of life
- Self-actualization
- Educational and career productivity
- Physical health

Affirmation: I want to have healthy relationships.

Exercise: Do you think you are a good listener? Honestly rate yourself as to your level of communication skills. Is there room for improvement?

_____

_____

_____

_____

_____

_____

_____

_____

_____

_____

_____

_____

_____

_____

_____

_____

SATURDAY

If you have already completed the previous six days this week, then this day is a free day to spend an hour doing something that you really love to do. If you haven't done the work, then today is your lucky day! Go for it. You will be so thankful you invested the time and energy into you! Enjoy a guided meditation.

Week Two

Week Two

Congratulations! You have completed the first week of your program and are about to begin the second. How did it go? What do you notice about yourself after week one? Are you starting to be a little kinder to your body? Are you finding it easy or difficult to find the 40 minutes each day for this practice? Is there anything different you need to try this week to make it easier? Remember, take it one day at a time. For today, simply make the firm commitment to be there for yourself for that 40 minutes tomorrow. And, then, tomorrow make the same commitment for the next day.

This week the theme is becoming more aware. Now, you might be wondering how and why you're going to do that, or you might think that you are already aware. The truth is, that most of us, most of the time, live in a state of selective awareness. We are aware of the things that support life the way we have it set up and we selectively hide from our awareness of the things that might rock the boat and cause change in our lives – if we were to be honest with ourselves. Think of your life of addiction or alcoholism. While in its hold, we don't truly allow ourselves to acknowledge the damage it does to our lives and our bodies. Yes, we know that it has a negative impact, but each time, we give into the addiction, we quickly push those thoughts away. We do not want that awareness of our consequences to get in the way of our relied upon habit.

Another big area of our lives in which we often put our awareness aside, is our relationships. Are we really conscious of what we are doing when we react to something our partner or family, and friends might say to us or do, or not do?

Awareness is the first step toward change. Without it, we usually remain static; without growth. Who's kidding whom? Becoming aware is tough. Coming into awareness, necessitates action. If we aren't aware, there is no need to change. Practicing awareness is not only about noticing the things you don't like. The beauty is that, it is also about noticing all the great moments in each day and having gratitude for these moments.

Practicing awareness demands that we slow our pace a little. If we are rushing from one thing to the next, we have little time to become aware of what is really happening in the moment.

For this week, we'll keep it simple. Try to focus your awareness on three areas: your body, your breath, and your thoughts. Check in with your body periodically during the day. How does it feel in the moment? How are you holding it? Where does it feel good and where does it not feel so good? How about your breath: is it deep and full, or shallow and rapid? And what are you thinking about? Check in with your mental process from time to time. Notice what seems to keep coming up during your day.

Focusing on your body, breath, and thoughts is also the concentration for your yoga and meditation practice this week. As you go through your 40 minute routine each day, bring your focus to the same three things during every part of it.

Body, breath, and thoughts; focus and intention setting

When you are ready to begin your practice, take two minutes to focus your attention on your body, your breath, and your thoughts; the activity of your mind. You can do this while sitting on the floor or standing, however you feel most comfortable at the time. Knowing that it is sometimes difficult to get started, I will often vary the position I use to begin. I allow myself to be in whatever position that feels good for the first few minutes of my focusing and intention setting.

After you have spent a few moments focusing on and noticing your body, do the same with your breath, and then, your thoughts. You don't have to do anything with what you notice. And, remember, this isn't time to think negatively of yourself.

After this, set your intention by asking yourself, "What is it I'm hoping to create in my life by doing this practice today?" With time, you will get used to this little daily exercise. It might seem simple; yet, it is very important. It's a way of connecting what we are doing to what we are wanting. And, we do this one day at a time. Notice that the question is about today, not next week or next year. Yes, those bigger and long-term intentions are also important, but for now, let's just look at today. What do you want to create in your life today and how will this time help you?

SUNDAY

Two Minutes
Body, Breath, and Thoughts – Focus and Intention Setting upon waking: focus on the day before you and the intention of your actions.

Thirty Minutes
20 push-ups: these can be wall push-ups, knee push-ups, or plank push-ups, as demonstrated in class. Key pointers: keep the back straight, not arched. Abdominals engaged and neck in neutral spine position.

20 ins and outs: these are great for the abdominals and core. You may have your hands on the ground or active in the exercise as well.

20 squats: key for your quads, core, and butt. Feet shoulder width apart, back straight, core engaged. Enjoy!

   – Take, at least, five 20-second awareness breaks today
   – Drink eight glasses of water today
   – Perform one small act today to support your intention of wellness
   – Schedule a treat for yourself, later this week
   – Let's do some yoga together! Grab your mat for yoga and meditation.

Journaling
This week you will record how your body is responding to the Mind-Body-Spirit program. Last week, you focused on what you were feeding your body. Hopefully, you became

increasingly aware of how your body responded to being treated with dignity through the feed you ate. This week you will record how your body is responding to its new program. How is your heart and mind responding to meditation? Is it challenging, calming, pleasant, troubling? Record it all. Be honest with yourself and express it on the page.

Today's thought…

Focus on living a quality life.

Put all the energy, emphasis, and willpower you used to spend on your addiction and alcoholism into the quality of your life.

It's key that you make yourself more important to you. Start with small things. A small act that shows you and others that you value you, even the act of sleeping in decent pajamas instead of an old ripped T-shirt. Indulge in long bubble baths. Eat better food. Get outside, go for a walk. Get in touch with someone you've been wanting to connect with, reach out!

You are worthy! Treat yourself as such. Commit yourself to living a quality life. Put all the energy, emphasis, and willpower you used to spend going on binges into increasing the quality of your life. Take advantage of all that is offered to you today. Don't miss a chance to experience beauty in the world and in you. Fill yourself with wonder, so you don't have to fill yourself with harmful substances. You deserve a quality life. Treat yourself with kindness and love.

Word for today: RELATIONSHIPS

While different types of relationships require varied attention, basically, they are all crucial to our well-being and wholeness. We all require certain relationships in our lives. Some, we wish we could avoid, while others, it seems, we can never get enough of.

Some people come into our lives and leave footprints on our hearts and we are never ever the same.

– Flavia Weeden

Affirmation: I now enjoy my own company; thereby, becoming an enjoyable companion.

Exercise: Describe below what kind of companion you have been and how you will be different now that you are becoming sober.

_____

_____

_____

_____

_____

_____

_____

_____

_____

_____

_____

_____

_____

_____

_____

_____

MONDAY

Two Minutes

Body, Breath, and Thoughts – Focus and Intention Setting upon waking. Focus on the day before you and the intention of your actions.

Twenty-Eight Minutes

20 push-ups: these can be wall push-ups, knee push-ups, or plank push-ups, as demonstrated in class. Key pointers: keep the back straight, not arched. Abdominals engaged and neck in neutral spine position.

20 ins and outs: these are great for the abdominals and core. You may have your hands on the ground or active in the exercise as well.

20 squats: key for your quads, core, and butt. Feet shoulder width apart, back straight, core engaged. Enjoy!

Journaling

This week you will record how your body is responding to the Mind-Body-Spirit program. Last week, you focused on what you were feeding your body. Hopefully, you became increasingly aware of how your body responded to being treated with dignity through the feed you ate. This week you will record how your body is responding to its new program. How is heart and mind responding to meditation? Is it challenging, calming, pleasant, troubling? Record it all. Be honest with yourself and the page.

– Take, at least, five 20-second awareness breaks today
– Drink eight glasses of water today
– Perform one small act today to support your intention of wellness
– Schedule a treat for yourself, later this week
– Is yoga time. Woot! Let's do it. Don't forget the guided meditation!

Today's thought:

Meditate.

When we're told that meditation can be a key part to our success, a first thought might be one of skepticism, "Yeah, sure it will help!" Do me a favour, park that skepticism and open your mind to its potential.

Quiet time is essential to give yourself perspective. Investing in five or ten minutes of silence every day, preferably in the morning, will help ensure your long-term success by keeping you connected to a source of power that lets your weary willpower off the hook. It will also keep you well grounded, more in charge of your life, and less afraid. Quiet time can include prayer, reading spiritual, or other uplifting literature, or writing in your journal, but meditation is the crux of it.

First, don't let the word meditation scare you. Meditation, which is sometimes called contemplation, is part of almost every religion on earth; and if you're not religious, you can meditate in a non religious way and still gain the mind, body, and spiritual benefits.

A simple way to begin to meditate on your own is to simply sit in a comfortable chair, close your eyes, and begin to notice how you are breathing. Pay attention to the air going into your nostrils and coming out again. This is simple meditation.

Next, you may begin to use a comforting phrase or words that you would like to guide your day. This could be something simple such as "happiness" on the inhalation and "contentment" on the exhalation. When words and thoughts enter your consciousness, simply let them go and resume the focus on the breath.

What you get in return for this simple practice is peace of mind, better health, a more positive attitude, and you'll tap into love! You also get a technique you can use when you need it, even for two or three minutes, anytime during the day when you need to improve your mood, calm yourself, regroup, or re-centre. Some days you will miss your meditation and that's okay. Just try not to miss too many. This is your gift to yourself; receive it.

Word for today: KINDNESS

Kindness consists of doing favours and good deeds for others, without the expectation of personal gain. Kindness is a type of strength that requires respect for others, but also includes emotional affection. Kind people find joy in the act of giving and helping other people, regardless of their degree of relatedness or similarity, without wanting anything in return.

This is my simple religion. There is no need for temples, no need for complicated philosophy. Our own brain, our own heart is our temple; the philosophy is kindness.

– The Dalai Lama

Affirmation: Kindness is its own reward.

Exercise: What is the kindest thing someone has done for you and what is the kindest thing you have ever done for someone else?

_____

_____

_____

_____

_____

_____

_____

_____

_____

_____

_____

_____

_____

_____

_____

_____

TUESDAY

Two Minutes

Body, Breath, and Thoughts – Focus and Intention Setting upon waking. Focus on the day before you and the intention of your actions.

Twenty-Eight Minutes

20 push-ups – these can be wall push-ups, knee push-ups, or plank push-ups, as demonstrated in class. Key pointers: keep the back straight, not arched. Abdominals engaged and neck in neutral spine position.

20 ins and outs – these are great for the abdominals and core. You may have your hands on the ground or active in the exercise as well.

20 squats – key for your quads, core, and butt. Feet shoulder width apart, back straight, and core engaged. Enjoy!

Journaling

This week you will record how your body is responding to the Mind-Body-Spirit program. Last week, you focused on what you were feeding your body. Hopefully, you became increasingly aware of how your body responded to being treated with dignity through the feed you ate. This week, you will record how your body is responding to its new program. How is heart and mind responding to meditation? Is it challenging, calming, pleasant, troubling? Record it all. Be honest with yourself and the page.

– Take, at least, five 20-second awareness breaks today
– Drink eight glasses of water today
– Perform one small act today to support your intention of wellness
– Schedule a treat for yourself, later this week
– It's time to meet on the mat. Let's do yoga! Welcome a guided meditation.

Today's thought…

Include an awareness of spirit.

If you feel that you deserve a better life to the one that you are currently living, please open your mind to the possibility that an awareness of spirit may have been something previously missing in your life. In fact, coming to a state of Mind-Body-Spirit wellness is what separates periods of sobriety from a life of wellness.

One way to see the spiritual component aspects in this is to realize that there is more to who you are than your body, intellect, and emotions. Your higher or deeper, or real self is that spiritual part of you; your essence. When you keep this in mind, you're more likely to live healthfully, because you value yourself more fully and you'll have something more than your human willpower to depend on.

How does that happen? When you begin to acknowledge your higher self, your self-worth develops, and intuitively guides you toward healthier, supportive practices. You begin to care for the one you care about. And now, for the first time in a long time, that person you are caring about is you!

Going deeper and having a spiritual component is absolutely necessary, if you believe you've done all you can to get a grip on your addiction and it keeps getting harder, and not easier, over time. If you can't do this yourself, give yourself a break and turn it over to something that can.

Including a spiritual component is simply knowing when you're up against something that is too much for you and your best intentions to handle on your own. It's realizing when you're weak and depending on something that is strong; whether you think of that as God in heaven or a power that, although, beyond your human ego, resides in yourself.

Word for today: GRIEF

Substance abuse treatment is a fertile field for dealing with the grief process. Patients and their families present for treatment, grieving the loss of the mood-altering substance, the loss of vitality, the loss of a family, the loss of employment, the loss of youth, the loss of self-respect, and for many, the loss of spirituality. But, few are aware of this. Like most, they don't associate substance abuse treatment with any form of grief.

— Kenneth A. Lucas. *A Buddhist Approach to Addiction, Grief and Psychotherapy.*

Think of it this way; our substance was our best "frenemy". It was always there for us – whatever the mood. Whatever the situation, we could always rely on our substance to be there with us, going through life with us. In some fucked-up way, we depended on our substance rather than depending on others to get us through life. But, where did it really leave us in the end?

It's normal to fear what life will be like without it. How could you not have fear? For so long, this "thing" has been your steadfast companion, your partner in crime. Your substance became part of you and came to define you. Take away the substance, what does that leave? It can be really hard to even remember what you were truly like before all of this started.

Be kind to yourself. You are not failing because you worry how you will get by clean and sober. It is normal to worry and to be afraid. Actually, this is a necessary stage of the journey. Just trust and know you will develop new patterns, new strategies, new coping skills, and real relationships that support and nurture you, rather than deplete you, your mind, body, and spirit.

Affirmation: I now choose the simple pleasures of everyday living.

Exercise: Write an epitaph for your addiction with all your feelings and memories, both, good and bad. Create a meaningful funeral for your addiction. Please allow yourself to experience all of the emotions this brings up for you. This is a powerful process.

_____

_____

_____

_____

_____

_____

_____

_____

_____

_____

_____

_____

_____

WEDNESDAY

Two Minutes

Body, Breath, and Thoughts – Focus and Intention Setting upon waking: focus on the day before you and the intention of your actions.

Twenty-Eight Minutes

20 push-ups – these can be wall push-ups, knee push-ups, or plank push-ups, as demonstrated in class. Key pointers: keep the back straight, not arched. Abdominals engaged and neck in neutral spine position.

20 ins and outs – these are great for the abdominals and core. You may have your hands on the ground or active in the exercise as well.

20 squats – key for your quads, core, and butt. Feet shoulder width apart, back straight, and core engaged. Enjoy!

Journaling

This week you will record how your body is responding to the Mind-Body-Spirit program. Last week, you focused on what you were feeding your body. Hopefully, you became increasingly aware of how your body responded to being treated with dignity through the feed you ate. This week, you will record how your body is responding to its new program. How is heart and mind responding to meditation? Is it challenging, calming, pleasant, troubling? Record it all. Be honest with yourself and the page.

- Take, at least, five 20-second awareness breaks today
- Drink eight glasses of water today
- Even if you really don't feel up to it today, get into some comfy clothing and let's do our yoga together. Enjoy a guided meditation.
- Perform one small act today to support your intention of wellness
- Schedule a treat for yourself, later this week

Today's thought...

Stay centered in today.

It's dangerous to get caught up in making promises to yourself about the future – committing to positive changes when certain things happen, or on certain days, or on a certain milestone. While it's great to plan and set goals for yourself, there can be a danger in failing to make the leap. This is the day you've got. No matter how praiseworthy your journaling and yoga and groups are, real change takes place with time. Small changes will add up. They will create a significant change in your life, but it is essential that you just stay in today.

Staying centered in the now keeps you focused on what you are doing. When you stay focused, you fully experience the day, its events, its sensations, and your growth. Life will become richer and more gratifying. You will worry less because worry is about the future and when the future becomes the present, it won't be nearly as frightening.

An added incentive for staying in today is that, this is where everything is happening: life, pleasure, accomplishment. Today is life. Today is your moment.

Word for today: MEDITATION

We now realize that it (meditation) activates the prefrontal cortex; the seat of higher thinking. It stimulates the release of neurotransmitters, including dopamine, serotonin, oxytocin, and brain opiates. Each of these naturally occurring brain chemicals has been linked to different aspects of happiness. Dopamine is an antidepressant, serotonin is associated with increased self-esteem, and Oxytocin is now believed to be the pleasant hormone, and opiates, and the body's painkillers. No single drug can simultaneously choreograph the coordinated release of all of these chemicals.

– Deepak Chopra, *The Ultimate Happiness Prescription*

Our culture and society is very materialistic and has emphasized and encouraged achieving satisfaction through external recognition, acquiring goods, and material pursuits, all of which only bring temporary pleasure but fail to fill an inner void. Addicted people, in particular, are apt to get fixated on external sources and quick fixes of comfort, excitement, and escape.

Meditation works because it teaches people to replace a destructive form of pleasure for another; a wholly constructive one. Specifically, becoming mindful is one of the most powerful benefits of meditation, along with reconnecting with one's inner self, learning to be comfortable in stillness, and reclaiming the ability to unwind in a natural way.

Affirmation: I find peace within.

Exercise: Choose to dedicate ten minutes every morning and every night to breathing deeply and calmly, while repeating the above affirmation, "I find peace within".

_____

_____

_____

_____

_____

_____

_____

_____

_____

_____

_____

_____

_____

_____

_____

THURSDAY

Two Minutes

Body, Breath, and Thoughts – Focus and Intention Setting upon waking. Focus on the day before you and the intention of your actions.

Twenty-Eight Minutes

20 push-ups – these can be wall push-ups, knee push-ups, or plank push-ups, as demonstrated in class.

Key pointers – keep the back straight, not arched, abdominals engaged, and neck in neutral spine position.

20 ins and outs – these are great for the abdominals and core. You may have your hands on the ground or active in the exercise as well.

20 squats – key for your quads, core, and butt! Feet shoulder width apart, back straight, and core engaged. Enjoy!

Journaling

This week you will record how your body is responding to the Mind-Body-Spirit program. Last week, you focused on what you were feeding your body. Hopefully, you became increasingly aware of how your body responded to being treated with dignity through the feed you ate. This week, you will record how your body is responding to its new program. How is heart and mind responding to meditation? Is it challenging, calming, pleasant, troubling? Record it all. Be honest with yourself and the page.

– Take, at least, five 20-second awareness breaks today
– Drink eight glasses of water today
– Smile! It's time for yoga. :) Enjoy a guided meditation.
– Perform one small act today to support your intention of wellness
– Schedule a treat for yourself, later this week

Today's thought…

Just keep moving forward.

Changing from the inside out requires changes in both lifestyle and personality. This is why it is important to consider all aspects of your being. How you see yourself, how you relate to the world around you, how much help you are willing to accept from your support network, and from whatever Higher Power is part of your sense of things.

In spite of all these aspects coming together for change, the only thing you have to concern yourself with today is, moving forward. Even if it sometimes involves taking a step back to just be. Do whatever you need to do to make sure you stay on your path to wellness. You do not have to be overwhelmed with thinking about forever. Today is enough.

Use the techniques you've learned from our weeks together. Keep this book and turn to your resources and supports, whenever you need them. Know that you can pull them out and read the parts that you need. You are working hard to bring yourself and your life into harmony. Honour that!

Remember, perfection does not exist in this world and sometimes, you will struggle. This program does not prevent life from happening. You will continue to live, laugh, and even, hurt. This is part of the process. Set reasonable parameters for yourself. Go into this day with the honest intention of contentment, moving forward, and not dwelling on past wrongs. Just keep moving forward!

Word for today: RECOVERY

I believe that if we are truly to recover from the disease of addiction, we must grow emotionally. True recovery is the product of humility that emerges from living and practicing a conscious and spiritual life. In order to attain humility, we must be honest with ourselves. This necessarily includes looking at the stupid things we do; today, or in recovery. I use the term "stupid" to indicate the things we do that are self-destructive and not in our best interest.

– Allen Berger, *12 Stupid things that Mess Up Recovery*

Recovery is the first step for the rest of our lives. We have the ultimate freedom of choice and it is important to begin with this understanding. We are not victims, regardless of how powerless we felt in the depths of addiction. You now have reclaimed your life, honour your power to make this choice permanent. Recovery is always your choice!

Affirmation: I choose recovery.

Exercise: Remind yourself of all of the good reasons you have chosen to be present.

_____

_____

_____

_____

_____

_____

_____

_____

_____

_____

_____

_____

_____

_____

_____

FRIDAY

Two Minutes

Body, Breath and Thoughts – Focus and Intention Setting upon waking: focus on the day before you and the intention of your actions.

Twenty-Eight Minutes

20 push-ups – these can be wall push-ups, knee push-ups, or plank push-ups, as demonstrated in class. Key pointers: keep the back straight, not arched. Abdominals engaged and neck in neutral spine position.

20 ins and outs – these are great for the abdominals and core. You may have your hands on the ground or active in the exercise as well.

20 squats – key for your quads, core, and butt. Feet shoulder width apart, back straight, and core engaged. Enjoy!

Journaling

This week you will record how your body is responding to the Mind-Body-Spirit program. Last week, you focused on what you were feeding your body. Hopefully, you became increasingly aware of how your body responded to being treated with dignity through the feed you ate. This week, you will record how your body is responding to its new program. How is heart and mind responding to meditation? Is it challenging, calming, pleasant, troubling? Record it all. Be honest with yourself and the page.

– Take, at least, five 20-second awareness breaks today
– Drink eight glasses of water today
– Bring all you have to your yoga practice today! Enjoy a guided meditation!
– Perform one small act today to support your intention of wellness
– Schedule a treat for yourself, later this week

Today's thought…

Give your senses something to do.

Our senses help keep us alive and help us appreciate that we are in the here and now. We need to nurture our senses by taking the time to appreciate the beauty and richness all around us, in its many forms. Take a few moments to feel blessed when taking in a beautiful sunset, the sound of laughter, or of the loving hug of a friend.

Eyes like looking at beauty, colour, and the passing joys of life. Ears like hearing lovely music, lyrical words, and the voices of people who care for them. Skin and nerve endings and the muscles underneath long for touch and stimulation. The olfactory nerves that detect smells also carry us back to some of the best moments of our life.

When living under the haze of substance abuse, our senses become dulled, not fully alive. Things don't taste the same. Music is a background noise. Movies and television are distractions. As the days progress, take time to reawaken your senses. Look at the colours that surround you. Enjoy the smells coming from the kitchen, where your meals are carefully prepared. Allow your muscles to come alive during yoga. Sink into the sounds of your early morning body, breath, and thoughts.

Indulge in all of your senses.

Word for today: SELF-ESTEEM

True self-esteem is not the same thing as improving your self-image. Self-image results from what other people think of you. The true self lies beyond images. It can be found at a level of existence that is independent of the good and bad opinions of others. It is fearless. It has infinite worth. When you shift your identity form, your self-image to your true self, you will find happiness that no one can take away from you.

 — Deepak Chopra, *The Ultimate Happiness Prescription*

Self-esteem is earned through our thoughts, words, and deeds. It is not easy to learn to value our true self, based on who we are, rather than what we have or do. The enduring qualities and virtues of a life well lived are created and we have the ability to create them. If you were blessed with good parents that helped create within you a healthy sense of self-worth, that's wonderful. But, it's only as adults that we can decide if we like the person looking back in the mirror. The truth will always come back from that deep place within; that inner self that cannot lie, no matter how hard our ego tries to practice self-deception.

Affirmation: I will strive to honor my true self.

Exercise: Imagine what you will feel when you feel good about yourself. How would your life be different?

_____

_____

_____

_____

_____

_____

_____

_____

_____

_____

_____

_____

_____

_____

_____

SATURDAY

If you have already completed the previous six days this week, then this day is a free day to spend an hour doing something that you really love to do, that supports your intention for being healthy, happy, and present. If you've missed a day, why don't you honour yourself and hunker down and do it! You are so worth it! Enjoy a guided meditation.

Week Three

Week Three

The theme for this week is acceptance. Last week, we practiced becoming more aware. Now, it's time to learn how to accept whatever awareness come to us.

Practicing acceptance does not mean that you are surrendering to the status quo and are not going to change anything. It simply means you are accepting what is, opening your heart, and mind to change. The steps of becoming aware and then, learning to accept what we have discovered about ourselves, is often not part of life's process. These steps take both time and self-inquiry. It's easier to skip these steps and rush for the first possible solution that appears. Or maybe, we don't even slow down enough to develop awareness; we just keep going, full speed ahead, hoping for change, but never doing the work to make change happen. I'm asking you to avoid the need to find a solution immediately. Stop rushing and trust in universe. Have acceptance in whatever you discover about yourself on this journey.

What if I Can't Accept?

You may have already asked that question and if you haven't, I can assure you that if you follow the guidance on practicing acceptance this week, there will be times when doubts arise. You will probably come across a particular awareness that you don't feel you can accept or even, just let be. What do you do with that? Well, the answer is simple, kind of! Just notice yourself not being able to accept. That is part of your reality, part of your awareness of self, and like everything else, it can be accepted, also.

Your program this week is similar to what you did last week with a few minor variations to fit the theme of acceptance.

Noticing and Accepting – Focus and Intention Setting

This week, as you begin your daily practice, take a few minutes to focus on acceptance. Do this by first focusing on your body, noticing, and accepting it just the way it is. Do the same with your breath and whatever else you are noticing about yourself, as you begin your practice. Also, take a moment to bring to your awareness what it is you want to create in your life by spending this time today to set your intention.

Meditation

Use our meditation this week to practice acceptance. Accept any thought you notice.

Accept any drifting into your past or future. A little trick you can use to help with practicing acceptance as you meditate is to notice and then, simply say to yourself...*and it is so* and exhale as you do.

Journaling

This week, make the focus of your journal, writing your awareness of yourself around the theme of acceptance: What can I accept about myself? What is difficult to accept? What guidance did I receive about this and how might it apply to my life?

Record anything else of importance that you notice, either during your practice or in the rest of your day.

Awareness Breaks

During the day this week and in subsequent weeks, you are asked to take some 20-second awareness breaks. An awareness break is simply stopping what you are doing or thinking, or saying and being still for 20 seconds and using those 20 seconds to notice what is happening to you and around you.

SUNDAY

Two Minutes
Notice and Accepting – Focus and Intention Setting

20 push-ups – these can be wall push-ups, knee push-ups, or plank push-ups. Key pointers: keep the back straights, not arched. Abdominals engaged and neck in neutral spine position.

20 ins and outs – these are great for the abdominals and core. You may have your hands on the ground or active in the exercise as well.

20 squats – key for your squads, core, and butt. Feet shoulder width apart, back straight, and core engaged. Enjoy!

– Take, at least, five 20-second awareness breaks today
– Practice accepting all that you notice
– Perform one small act to support your intention
– Schedule a treat for your body, later this week
– Drink eight glasses of water today

Yoga practice and guided meditation:
– Pop in the yoga DVD and enjoy! Proud of you. Enjoy a guided meditation.

Today's thought…
Deal with your stress.

This is your opportunity to learn new methods for dealing with life's stressors. There are tons of ways to reduce stress and hopefully, we'll explore ways to do that together – and find something that works for you! Learning yoga and meditation, getting regular exercise, seeing a therapist, and looking more closely at what spirituality has to offer, are all great stress reduction techniques. So is keeping a journal and talking about problems, and decide to spend time with someone who will listen more than talk.

There are other techniques that can be readily used. The easiest and most available technique is breathing. We've already explored breathing in the previous weeks, but it is such a simple, effective tool that I wanted to go over it again. Slow, deep breathing; in through your nose, out through your mouth. This technique can calm you down when you are anxious or angry. A hot bath will work. Self-massage; kneading the kinks out of your shoulder, neck, and hands can help reduce tension. A change of scene; go outside, if you're inside, lie down, if you're up, or take a walk, if you are stewing on the couch. Begin to recognize which situations cause stress in your life and can be triggers to relapse. Recognizing these situations goes a long way in both, preventing and managing your life and having more control, and ownership.

Your substance is what you used to use to get you through or avoid experiencing stress. Now, you have to figure out how to get through the tough times, without something that may have served you for a long time. You need to replace it with other tools. This is incredibly challenging, I'm not going to sugar coat it for you. If you are willing to try to begin to deal with stress in healthy ways, you will eventually live a life fuller and happier than your life while using ever did. You will have a healthier life, full of wellness.

Word for today: SELF-DISCOVERY

When you take the first step towards self-development, many doors of friendship and happiness will be opened for you.

Many addictions are caused by the fear of one's own inner self. We do not want to deal with painful or uncomfortable emotions, so we try to suppress, ignore, drown, or change the way we feel through substances. We now know that doesn't work!

Self-discovery is turning our attention inwards and having the courage to explore our inner world. This is no small feat, because it's unchartered territory with no map to guide us.

So, what exactly does self-discovery mean? Self-discovery means paying attention and discovering who you are. Self-discovery means that we are responsible for being aware of our needs and how to nurture our true self.

Affirmation: I am now willing to embark on the voyage of self-discovery.

Exercise: Talk about yourself in the space below. Start simple; write down what you do know about yourself, such as your taste in music, favorite food, recreational activities that give you pleasure; movies, playing sports, creative crafts, which season do you prefer. Continue to explore you. What makes you happy? What makes you sad? What brings you joy?

_____

_____

_____

_____

_____

_____

_____

_____

_____

_____

_____

_____

_____

_____

MONDAY

Two Minutes

Notice and Accepting – Focus and Intention Setting

20 push-ups – these can be wall push-ups, knee push-ups, or plank push-ups. Key pointers: keep the back straights, not arched. Abdominals engaged and neck in neutral spine position.

20 ins and outs – these are great for the abdominals and core. You may have your hands on the ground or active in the exercise as well.

20 squats – key for your squads, core, and butt. Feet shoulder width apart, back straight, and core engaged. Enjoy!

– Take, at least, five 20-second awareness breaks today
– Practice accepting all that you notice
– Perform one small act to support your intention
– Schedule a treat for your body, later this week
– Drink eight glasses of water today

Yoga practice and guided meditation:
–   Pop in the yoga DVD and enjoy! Proud of you. Enjoy a guided meditation.

Today's thought...

Be kind to yourself on difficult days.

Everyone has to deal with bad days. You get through them by going through them. The challenge for someone struggling to maintain sobriety is how to get through bad days, without giving into the temptation to use. To do this, you first have to resign yourself to the fact that difficult days are normal and happen to every person on earth, even people who seem like they're living the dream.

The next step is to remind yourself as often as necessary that, in almost every case, shitty times are temporary. It's really normal when you're at this point, to see every difficulty as permanent. Don't worry, you're not alone in feeling this way. To keep from relapsing, it is important that you recognize the difference between a bad day and a futile life. Once you realize you are having a bad day or two, you can take a moment and give yourself a break, cut yourself some slack, and treat yourself to an act of kindness. This is when you need to learn to be gentle with yourself and practice this gentleness, when it means the most.

It is also important to acknowledge that we may have more than one bad day. During stretches that seem really rough, you have to intentionally put something bright into each day. This is tough to do, especially if you think it would feel better being miserable. This is easier said than done, I know. But, I promise that if you make the effort to support yourself with kindness, it will be returned to you tenfold.

Spiritual readings are likely to speak to you more clearly now than at any other time. You'll even find new insights in readings familiar to you. If you feel you are in real trouble, you need to seek out someone; a counselor, a spiritual leader, whoever and acknowledge your struggles, without losing sight of all that is full of hope and goodness.

Word for today: FREEDOM

Liberty, autonomy, lack of restrictions, self-determination, independence, choice, and free will are some of the synonyms for this wondrous state of being. You are now well into your own freedom from the chains of the addiction, which were controlling your life.

History shows how fiercely we fight to be free. Countless brave people have sacrificed their lives in the name of freedom. Are you willing to sacrifice your freedom, anymore?

Freedom is nothing else but a chance to be better.
— Albert Camus

No man is free, who in not a master of himself.

— Epicteus

The basic test of freedom is perhaps less in what we are free to do than in what we are not free to do.

— Eric Hoffler

Affirmation: I have the courage to fight for my freedom from addiction.

Exercise: Describe how it's beginning to feel as you become free of your addiction. Describe the battles it took to make this decision.

_____

_____

_____

_____

_____

_____

_____

_____

_____

_____

_____

_____

_____

_____

_____

_____

TUESDAY

Two Minutes

Notice and Accepting – Focus and Intention Setting

20 push-ups – these can be wall push-ups, knee push-ups, or plank push-ups. Key pointers: keep the back straights, not arched. Abdominals engaged and neck in neutral spine position.

20 ins and outs – these are great for the abdominals and core. You may have your hands on the ground or active in the exercise as well.

20 squats – key for your squads, core, and butt. Feet shoulder width apart, back straight, and core engaged. Enjoy!

– Take, at least, five 20-second awareness breaks today
– Practice accepting all that you notice
– Perform one small act to support your intention
– Schedule a treat for your body, later this week
– Drink eight glasses of water today

Yoga practice and guided meditation:
Pop in the yoga DVD and enjoy! Proud of you.

Today's thought...

Develop an attitude of gratitude.

Have an attitude of gratitude. Without an attitude of gratitude, renewable every day, you leave yourself open to negativity and that is often the first step to relapse.

Acknowledging your blessings with gratitude is key in preventing relapse.

A helpful exercise is to write ten things you're grateful for every day, in your journaling. If you get discouraged, frustrated, or overwhelmed during the day, write ten more. Big things, little things; it doesn't matter. They can even be the same ten things every day.

Once you acknowledge and write your ten gratitudes, your day looks different. Your life feels better. Your world seems more accommodating. On tough mornings, the ones when getting out of bed seems like a bad idea, you may want to make your list mentally before your feet touch the floor. It can get your priorities in order, almost instantly.

When gratitude moves in, happiness usually comes along. If you start every day by making a gratitude list, whether on paper or in your mind and heart, you are consciously aware that you are living a life worthy of gratitude and life becomes that much sweeter.

You are, then, able to acknowledge the good things that happen to you, during your day. Things you may have overlooked before now, become blessings. You'll notice beauty you might have overlooked before. Eventually, you will find it hard to keep your list to ten gratitudes.

Word for today: FOCUS

How often has someone said to you, "Would you, please, just focus?"

How do we train ourselves to remain focused on one subject at a time?

The technique is simple and it is known as mindfulness. Pay attention to the present moment. Be mindful of everything around you and most importantly, stop time traveling in your mind. The majority of people are living in the past, thinking about the future, scattered everywhere in their mind, except in the only place that truly exists; this present moment. Focus is constantly correcting your course, staying in the present moment, and taking good care of what is before you.

Your brain is just like a muscle. You are able to exercise being in the moment with practice and mindfulness.

Affirmation: I am mindful. I am focused.

Exercise: An excellent tool in retraining your mind is learning to memorize something simple. It allows you to concentrate and focus your attention on the present. Try to memorize the saying below. Give it a shot:

> We are what we think. All that we are arises with our thoughts. With our thoughts, we make our world.
> — Buddha

Try to write about how easy or difficult it was to memorize this passage. Let the value of focus, begin to be appreciated.

_____

_____

_____

_____

_____

_____

_____

_____

_____

_____

_____

_____

WEDNESDAY

Two Minutes

Notice and Accepting – Focus and Intention Setting

20 push-ups – these can be wall push-ups, knee push-ups, or plank push-ups. Key pointers: keep the back straights, not arched. Abdominals engaged and neck in neutral spine position.

20 ins and outs – these are great for the abdominals and core. You may have your hands on the ground or active in the exercise as well.

20 squats – key for your squads, core, and butt. Feet shoulder width apart, back straight, and core engaged. Enjoy!

– Take, at least, five 20-second awareness breaks today
   – Practice accepting all that you notice
   – Perform one small act to support your intention
   – Schedule a treat for your body, later this week
   – Drink eight glasses of water today

Yoga practice and guided meditation:
– Simply release…
   – Pop in the yoga DVD and enjoy! Proud of you.

Today's thought…

Just keep moving forward.

Changing from the inside means making changes in both how you live and think. This is why I encourage you to explore the many varied and rich aspects of your being. How you see yourself, how you relate to the world around you, and how much help you are willing to accept from whatever High Power is part of your sense of things. You will realize you are more than the person you were tied to a substance, living in a world of negative thoughts and behaviours.

Even when all of these aspects are coming together to change your body and your life, the only thing you have to concern yourself with today is moving forward. Do whatever you need to do to keep from relapsing. Do not think in terms of tomorrow or forever. Today is enough. Use techniques you are learning. Be fearless in your desire to succeed by reaching out to those who will help you. You can expect to get what you need, including the necessary degree of transformation to make the most of your life. Perfection does not exist in this world and sometimes, you will be tempted to use. You will crave. You will remember using almost romantically. This is part of the process. It's how you learn that your life is clean enough. Your clean life has value and meaning. Go into this day with the honest intention of staying clean. Keep moving forward today and leave the past behind.

Word for the day: PATIENCE

One moment of patience may ward off great disaster.
One moment of impatience may ruin a whole life.
— Chinese proverb

Patience is also a form of action.
— August Robin

Adopt the pace of nature; her secret is patience.
— Ralph Waldo Emerson

Affirmation: Patience is waiting, not passively waiting; that is laziness. But to keep going when the going is hard and slow, that is patience.

Exercise: Explore how patience is essential in recovery. How has not having patience derailed you in the past?

_____

_____

_____

_____

_____

_____

_____

_____

_____

_____

_____

_____

_____

_____

_____

_____

THURSDAY

Two Minutes

Notice and Accepting – Focus and Intention Setting

20 push-ups – these can be wall push-ups, knee push-ups, or plank push-ups. Key pointers: keep the back straights, not arched. Abdominals engaged and neck in neutral spine position.

20 ins and outs – these are great for the abdominals and core. You may have your hands on the ground or active in the exercise as well.

20 squats – key for your squads, core, and butt. Feet shoulder width apart, back straight, and core engaged. Enjoy!

- Take, at least, five 20-second awareness breaks today
  - Practice accepting all that you notice
  - Perform one small act to support your intention
  - Schedule a treat for your body, later this week
  - Drink eight glasses of water today

Yoga practice and guided meditation, relax and breathe.
- Pop in the yoga DVD and enjoy! Proud of you.

Today's thought...

Make peace with your past and other people.

The past is over, but it is not necessarily done with. Until it is, it can lead to a return of addiction and abuse. Wading in old hurts and disappointments is never easy, but without being willing to face the deep-seated issues that may be responsible or contributing to your addiction, you may be keeping yourself in a vulnerable place and risking relapse.

An effective way to make peace is to forgive the people who harmed you and forgive yourself for your own mistakes. You deal with the instances in which you feel you were at fault by showing up and setting things right to the degree that you can and then, you have to let it go. If letting go is hard for you, keep at it. It's hard for everybody, but it is essential to your recovery.

When someone has hurt you, forgiveness can be challenging. On the other hand, forgiveness is not saying, "It's okay that you were terrible to me. You can do it again." Rather, it's realizing that hurt comes from hurt. Forgiveness releases the person to their own fate and frees you from the old hurts. This is equally important if you're in need of forgiving yourself from harm you have caused yourself and others. This is as much for you, as for the other person. You need the weight of what happened lifted from your heart and mind. What you have done does not define who you are. At your core, you are truly a source of light and love.

Do the work that needs to be done. Seek out the help and guidance you need from a friend, family member, professional, or spiritual mentor. The guidance of someone else may enable you to experience a series of 'Aha! Moments', so things that never made sense before, can start becoming clear.

Value yourself and this process enough to make peace with yourself and others.

Word for today: INNER WISDOM

Where does wisdom come from? Wisdom speaks from all corners of our world and age is not always a factor. Wisdom comes from a calm knowingness, life experience, a clear and sober mind, and an ability to see the bigger picture.

Understanding, knowledge, insight, perception, astuteness, intelligence, acumen, and good judgment are all synonyms for wisdom. Your decision to begin the journey to sobriety is a wise decision. You have wisdom within you. Do not lose sight of this and listen to your inner voice, your inner truth. Begin to trust this inner voice, your inner wisdom. It is your guide.

Affirmation: I now choose to cultivate wisdom in all life choices.

Exercise: Think carefully of all the times you have made a wise decision and list the benefits you enjoyed from this.

_____

_____

_____

_____

_____

_____

_____

_____

_____

_____

_____

_____

_____

_____

_____

_____

131

FRIDAY

Two Minutes

Notice and Accepting – Focus and Intention Setting

20 push-ups – these can be wall push-ups, knee push-ups, or plank push-ups. Key pointers: keep the back straights, not arched. Abdominals engaged and neck in neutral spine position.

20 ins and outs – these are great for the abdominals and core. You may have your hands on the ground or active in the exercise as well.

20 squats – key for your squads, core, and butt. Feet shoulder width apart, back straight, and core engaged. Enjoy!

- Take, at least, five 20-second awareness breaks today
- Practice accepting all that you notice
- Perform one small act to support your intention
- Schedule a treat for your body, later this week
- Drink eight glasses of water today

Yoga practice and guided meditation; just breathe.
- Pop in the yoga DVD and enjoy! Proud of you.

Today's thought...

It's all going to be okay. Our challenging times are preparing us for the next great thing.

One thing I can come to truly believe, is that when we are going through truly shitty times, the universe is readying us for the next phase we are about to enter. Having that knowing is both a comfort and a blessing. I still have times in my life when I disappoint myself tremendously or relationships are experiencing true hardships. But now, I am able to actually step back and know the hardships will pass.

You don't have to appear as though you have it all under control, every minute of the day. Refusing to worry about what you can do nothing about is essential. Do your best to be less distraught when things don't work out the way you'd hoped they would. More often than not, this means that life has something better in store for you, anyhow.

Sometimes, we just need to trust that our challenging periods happen to prepare and strengthen us for the good that is in store for us. When you begin to place your trust and hope in God and the universe, when you begin to believe it will all work out, even though you cannot see a possible way, you carry a light within you. It is the light of hope, goodness, and love and it radiates outwards. Your light instils hope in others and encourages them on their journey, through their struggles. And so, "lighten up" takes on a deeper and far richer meaning.

Word for today: COMPASSION

Most people think of compassion as a desired trait like, honesty, loyalty, or spontaneity. If you have compassion, you show it by being kind, sympathetic, and helpful to others. This is certainly true. But, compassion and its impact on self-esteem, is much more. First of all, it is not an unchanging character trait. Compassion is actually a skill; a skill that you can increase, if you lack it or improve it, if you already have it. And, compassion is not something you feel only for others. It should also inspire you to be kind, sympathetic, and helpful to yourself. There are three basic attributes that make up compassion: understanding, acceptance, and forgiveness.

Affirmation: As a compassionate person, I am now kind, sympathetic, and helpful to myself and to others.

Exercise: Write how learning the skill of compassion could change the way you treat yourself and others. Choose a good memory of when someone treated you with compassion and journal how that helped you.

_____

_____

_____

_____

_____

_____

_____

_____

_____

_____

_____

_____

_____

_____

SATURDAY

If you have already completed the previous six days this week, then this day is a free day to spend an hour doing something that you really love to do, which supports your recovery. If you're not where you want to be in this work, do it today! Meditate...

Week Four

Week Four

Okay, so, now, you're beginning to notice the benefits and changes of Mind Body Spirit. Hopefully, your body has begun to feel different because of the yoga practice and healthy eating. You'll also notice that your thinking and your way of being in the world is starting to shift. At first, the changes will be subtle and barely noticeable. Then, one day, you'll simply become aware of not doing the same things the same way, anymore.

So, if you haven't noticed too many changes, maybe you haven't been sticking with the program each day and that's okay! Be kind to yourself and don't stress about it. If this is you, what do you do? Do you quit? No way! Maybe, you want to recommit and start the program from where you left off. Maybe, you're the kind of person who wants to go back to week one and start over. The choice is yours. But, it's my true hope that you will just do it! Just open the book and read. Put the yoga DVD in and connect with your body. Listen to the meditation CD and simply be. Honour yourself. Love yourself. I would take some time and meditate on what you do next and where you re-immerse yourself in the program. It will become clear to you. The neat thing is that you can start again, anytime you want. With this book as your guide, you can do this on your terms. All I can tell you is that if you can just stay with it, you will reconnect with your mind, body, and spirit. This is your journey and my intention is to support you in your work.

We all make commitments we find it difficult to live up to from time to time, but if we know they are commitments that are in our best interest or ones we truly want to keep, we recommit. We start over and do what we originally intended to do. Just remember our goal when we started; to commit to one day at a time and it will all fall into place. You are worth it! Even if you have kept to the program, you may want to go back from time to time and revisit certain sections that you find encouraging and supportive, the ones that truly spoke to you. Each time you do, you'll get something new out of it. Believe it or not, you are blessed to be in a place where you have the choice to be doing mind, body, and spirit. What a gift to be present enough and well-enough to engage in yoga recovery. And, that is why the theme for this week is choice.

You know better than most that being able to be in a place where you can actually have choices, takes time. It starts with when you begin to become aware; aware of where you are at on your journey. Once you develop awareness, it is so important to be able to accept your awareness and to accept where you are. When we can see where we are at, we are then able to also see the choices that lay before us. Choices are available in every moment and in all we do – our thoughts, our actions, and even, our emotions. Part of the beauty of clean living is having the clarity of being in the moment, of being aware of our life, as we are living it. This "being in the moment" provides us with the opportunity to actively change our reality. We can choose our present moments. If our choices are not supporting us in creating what we want in our lives, then, maybe, we need to look at the choices we are making. Maybe we're making choices out of habit or choices because they're expedient – a choice for a few fleeting moments of pleasure, the promise of better things to come, but at the end, not for real happiness.

At the start of this program and each day, when you set your intention, you are making a statement to yourself about what you are really seeking in life. As you become more aware of your intention and goals, you can continue to do what you've done in the past or based on your new awareness, you can choose to do something different. You can choose something that will support a healthy life; mind, body, and spirit. It may not always be the easy choice but, when choices are made to support your intention of being present and healthy, they are always worth the effort. I promise!

Choice is powerful. It means we can move in new directions and bring about real change. Move slowly and carefully, begin with this one new change in your life. Take the time to feel the impact of this new choice, before making any more. What will be helpful in making the smaller day to day choices is becoming aware of the choices you are currently making. Part of your practice, this week, will be to discover your choices by being more aware, as you actively engage in each moment of the day. Remember, you are moving from a place of no choice to a place of infinite potential. In doing so, we become the victor, not the victim! How great is that? And, guess what? The power to choose to be victorious is all yours – you have the power within you!

SUNDAY

Two Minutes
Notice and Accepting – Focus and Intention Setting

Five Minutes
Meditation and Integration

– Take, at least, five 20-second awareness breaks today
– Practice accepting all that you notice
– Notice what you are currently choosing
– Drink eight glasses of water today
– Perform one small act to support your intention
– Schedule a treat for your body for later this week

20 push-ups – these can be wall push-ups, knee push-ups, or plank push-ups. Key pointers: keep the back straight, not arched. Abdominal engaged and neck in neutral spine position.

20 ins and outs – these are great for the abdominals and core. You may have your hands on the ground or active in the exercise as well.

20 squats – key for your quads, core, and butt. Feet should width apart, back straight, and core engaged. Enjoy!

– Do yoga with me, today! Enjoy a guided mediation.

Today's thought…

Affirming your choices.

You are standing in the corridor of Life and behind you, so many doors have closed.

Things you no longer do or say, or think. Experiences you no longer have. Ahead of you in an unending corridor of doors, each one opens to a new experience. As you move forward, see yourself opening various doors on wonderful experiences that you would like to have. Trust that your inner guide is leading you and guiding you in ways that are best for you and that your spiritual growth is continuously expanding. No matter which door opens or which door closes, you are always safe. You are eternal. You will go on, forever, from experience to experience. See yourself opening doors to joy, peace, healing, prosperity, and love, doors to understanding, compassion, and forgiveness. Doors to self-love. It is all here, before you. Which door will you open first?

Remember you are safe, this is only healing change.

Word for the day: CHANGE

The key to change...is to let go of fear.
— Rosanne Cash

All changes, even the most longed for, have their melancholy; for what we leave behind us, is a part of ourselves. We must die to one life before we can enter another.

— Anatole France

Any change, even a change for the better, is always accompanied by drawbacks and discomforts.

— Arnold Bennett

Affirmation: I now seek to find joy in all things life has given me.

Exercise: Describe what changes need to take place in order to live sober and happy in this moment, on this day.

_____

_____

_____

_____

_____

_____

_____

_____

_____

_____

_____

_____

_____

_____

_____

_____

MONDAY

Two Minutes
Notice and Accepting – Focus and Intention Setting

Five Minutes
Meditation and Integration

– Take, at least, five 20-second awareness breaks today
– Practice accepting all that you notice
– Notice what you are currently choosing
– Drink eight glasses of water today
– Perform one small act to support your intention
– Schedule a treat for your body for later this week

20 push-ups – these can be wall push-ups, knee push-ups, or plank push-ups. Key pointers: keep the back straight, not arched. Abdominal engaged and neck in neutral spine position.

20 ins and outs – these are great for the abdominals and core. You may have your hands on the ground or active in the exercise as well.

20 squats – key for your quads, core, and butt. Feet should width apart, back straight, and core engaged. Enjoy!

– Do yoga with me, today! Slip into a guided mediation.

Today's thought...
Do whatever it takes.

In the beginning and for as long as it takes, do whatever you have to do to keep yourself away from the sources of your addiction. Cravings will surface and when they do, you do not want to give into the temptation, due to easy access.

When this craving surfaces, take whatever action is called for. Phone a friend who can come to your side. Or, get out of yourself and think of others, call someone you know has been having a difficult time and ask how you can help. Turn the tables. Help yourself by helping another. You might play music as loud as possible; let the auditory stimulation jolt you back to clearer thinking. Take a bath. Visit somebody. Go see a movie. Go to a book store. Do yoga. Meditate. Pray. Play.

These are simple suggestions. You will find others to help you ride out the craving. When you don't give into it, a craving is a short-lived entity. Even the powerful ones that seem to overwhelm you. Rationalizing to yourself all of the reasons you should give in. Find the strength to resist. Remember how good you felt when you first became aware you were clean and feeling healthy. Remember how in those moments you never wanted to go back to using. These cravings will eventually stop…when they aren't fed. Ride them out often enough and they will get the message that there is no use in bothering you any longer.

Word for today: LOVE

Take away love and our earth is a tomb.
— Robert Browning

The kind of love that the greatest thinkers and saviours of the world talked about, is very different from what most people understand love to be. It is much more than loving your family, friends, and favourite things, because love is not just a feeling; love is a positive force! Love is not weak, feeble, or soft. Love is the positive force of life. Love is the cause of everything positive and good. There are not a hundred different positive forces in life. There is only one.
— Rhonda Bryne, *The Power*

Love is a state of consciousness. When you have love in your heart, there is no room for hate, cruelty, judgements, and criticisms. Love allows all of life to have their chance in the sun, from the smallest being in the different kingdoms of nature's life forms to all members of the human family. Love sees beauty where others see ugliness. Love honours nature and appreciates each day of life as a new opportunity to express love.

Love is full of laughter, joy, and wisdom. Love is the highest and best expression in us all.

Affirmation: Love is the cause of everything positive and good.

Exercise: Write of love – your memories, and experiences of what love feels like. Please, keep this exercise only positive; remember the goodness and happiness of love, while it has existed in your life.

_____

_____

_____

_____

_____

_____

_____

_____

_____

_____

_____

_____

_____

_____

_____

_____

TUESDAY

Two Minutes
Notice and Accepting – Focus and Intention Setting

Five Minutes
Meditation and Integration:

– Take, at least, five 20-second awareness breaks today
– Practice accepting all that you notice
– Notice what you are currently choosing
– Drink right glasses of water today
– Perform one small act to support your intention
– Schedule a treat for your body for later this week

20 push-ups: these can be wall push-ups, knee push-ups, or plank push-ups. Key pointers: keep the back straight, not arched. Abdominal engaged and neck in neutral spine position.

20 ins and outs: these are great for the abdominals and core. You may have your hands on the ground or active in the exercise as well.

20 squats: key for your quads, core, and butt. Feet should width apart, back straight, and core engaged. Enjoy!

– Do yoga with me, today! Simply be with a guided meditation.

Today's thought...
Stay centered in today.

Today is the day you've got. Do no set overwhelming goals for yourself. The tiny changes you are making each day will add up. Just stay in today.

When you live for today, you stay in the present. You live out the work of recovery. Today is it. What you do today is all that matters. Staying centered in the now keeps you aware of what you're doing. You will be far less likely to give into defeatist thoughts and behaviours. When you stay focused, you experience the day; its events, its sensations, its nuances. Life will become richer and more gratifying. You will have fewer regrets because regrets belong to the past. You will worry less because worry is about the future and when the future becomes the present, it won't be nearly as frightening. The present almost never is.

Keeping your focus on the here and now also makes it possible to live the way you desire. An incentive for staying in today is that this is where everything is happening; life, pleasure, accomplishment. Today is where it all happens and you are already here. Live it!

Word for today: FORGIVENESS

There are three essential parts to self-forgiveness:
1. Acknowledge having acted in the wrong and accepting responsibility for that wrong.
2. Allow yourself to experience feelings of guilt and regret.
3. And, finally, overcome these feelings through forgiveness and self-forgiveness, and in doing so, experience a motivational change away from self-punishment towards self-acceptance.

Forgiveness is giving up the idea of having a better past. I can forgive, but I cannot forget, is only another way of saying I will not forgive. Forgiveness ought to be like a cancelled note; torn in two and burned up, so that it can never be shown against one.
– Henry Ward Beecher

The weak can never forgive. Forgiveness is the attribute of the strong.
– Mahatma Gandhi

Affirmation: Forgiveness of myself and others sets me free form the past.

Exercise: Which experience lays heavy on your heart? Do you need to forgive yourself or someone else to restore peace within you? What stands in your way; is it pride, anger, righteousness, or stubbornness? Be honest with yourself, as you begin to explore the miraculous power of forgiveness.

_____

_____

_____

_____

_____

_____

_____

_____

_____

_____

_____

_____

_____

_____

WEDNESDAY

Two Minutes

Notice and Accepting – Focus and Intention Setting

Five Minutes

Meditation and Integration:

– Take, at least, five 20-second awareness breaks today
– Practice accepting all that you notice
– Notice, what you are currently choosing
– Drink eight glasses of water today
– Perform one small act to support your intention
– Schedule a treat for your body for later this week

20 push-ups – these can be wall push-ups, knee push-ups, or plank push-ups. Key pointers: keep the back straight, not arched. Abdominal engaged and neck in neutral spine position.

20 ins and outs – these are great for the abdominals and core. You may have your hands on the ground or active in the exercise as well.

20 squats – key for your quads, core, and butt. Feet should width apart, back straight, and core engaged. Enjoy!

Thank you for sharing your yoga practice with me today, Namaste! Enjoy the meditation!

Today's thought...

Never punish yourself.

There are all sorts of ways to punish yourself for your situation. A negative punishing attitude toward yourself won't help you in your goal to live a healthy, clean life. Instead, do the best you can. If you have fallen short, now is the time to begin again. Treat yourself with the love and kindness you would offer someone who is struggling and allow yourself the space to move forward. Getting through substance abuse and the journey of recovery can be challenging enough, without you being your own worst enemy. Love starts here, from within. Let the flicker of self-love grow from within, until it radiates outward. Simply allow yourself the room you need to grow and reach your fullness.

If you have been punitive and defeatist in the past, watch what you say to yourself, both, inside and outside your head. Watch for the subtle ways you punish yourself. Don't see yourself in terms of failure. Keep yourself in the safety of this day; this will help make setbacks less likely. When you disappoint yourself, treat yourself the way you would treat your best friend under similar circumstances.

Be a friend to yourself. Learn the lessons life presents. And, in the meantime, let yourself grow, heal, renew, rejuvenate, and triumph.

Word for today: RESPECT

To be respectful, is an attitude of caring for the feelings of others. To have self-respect means that you have become aware of how precious life is. A caring attitude towards oneself, others, and the earth demonstrates someone rooted in love, gratitude, and grace.

If you want to be respected by others, the great thing is to respect yourself. Only by that, only by self-respect, will you compel others to respect you.
– Fyodor Dostoyevsky

Affirmation: I, now, cultivate an understanding that all deserve respect, myself included.

Exercise: Remember a time you were treated with disrespect. Write what the word "respect" means to you and how you are cultivating this attitude within you.

_____

_____

_____

_____

_____

_____

_____

_____

_____

_____

_____

_____

_____

_____

_____

_____

_____

THURSDAY

Two Minutes
Notice and Accepting – Focus and Intention Setting

Five Minutes
Meditation and Integration:

– Take, at least, five 20-second awareness breaks today
– Practice accepting all that you notice
– Notice what you are currently choosing
– Drink eight glasses of water today
– Perform one small act to support your intention
– Schedule a treat for your body for later this week

20 push-ups –these can be wall push-ups, knee push-ups, or plank push-ups. Key pointers: keep the back straight, not arched. Abdominal engaged and neck in neutral spine position.

20 ins and outs – these are great for the abdominals and core. You may have your hands on the ground or active in the exercise as well.

20 squats – key for your quads, core, and butt. Feet shoulder width apart, back straight, and core engaged. Enjoy!

– Enjoy the bliss yoga offers. Let it all go with a guided meditation.

Today's thought...
Tap into your courage.

Courage is not reserved for those who save lives or make headlines. We all have courage. We have the potential to live with courage in our everyday lives. The courage you need for most days is subtle. It is the courage that allows you to abstain from addiction. It is the courage that allows you to be present in your life, your family, your marriage, or your place of work. It is the courage to smile, when you're struggling the most.

Courage is an odd quality in that you may have a great deal of it in one area and virtually, none in another. You may have no idea how brave you are, until you are facing your first challenge or trigger. In recovery, the greatest courage you can demonstrate is the ability to say no, to walk away, and abstain. It takes courage to put yourself out there, trust in others, and develop new relationships that are healthy and supportive. It can create fears, for sure. Reduce fear by taking each day as it comes. Deal with various stressors (relationships, overscheduling, finances) and be so good to yourself on the ordinary days that you'll be up to the challenge of difficult days.

Whether you feel you need more courage to deal with recovery or with other issues, calling upon your higher power will strengthen your resolve. When you're counting on your higher power or a higher purpose, you've got a light to help you through the dark places.

Word for the day: TOLERANCE

Surely, the day will come when colour means nothing more than skin tone, when religion is seen uniquely as a way to speak one's soul, when birth places have the weight of a throw of a dice, and all men are born free, when understanding breeds love and brotherhood.

– Josephine Baker

It is, thus, tolerance that is the source of peace and intolerance, that is, the source of disorder and squabbling.

– Peter Bayle

Affirmation: I now seek to practice tolerance by understanding myself and others.

Exercise: In the practice of tolerance, one's enemy is the best teacher.

— 14th Dalai Lama.

Think of a person that has helped you learn the lesson of tolerance. What was the lesson? How did this help you grow?

_____

_____

_____

_____

_____

_____

_____

_____

_____

_____

_____

_____

_____

_____

FRIDAY

Two Minutes

Notice and Accepting – Focus and Intention Setting

Five Minutes

Meditation and Integration:

– Take, at least, five 20-second awareness breaks today
– Practice accepting all that you notice
– Notice what you are currently choosing
– Drink eight glasses of water today
– Perform one small act to support your intention
– Schedule a treat for your body for later this week

20 push-ups – these can be wall push-ups, knee push-ups, or plank push-ups. Key pointers: keep the back straight, not arched, abdominal engaged, and neck in neutral spine position.

20 ins and outs – these are great for the abdominals and core. You may have your hands on the ground or active in the exercise as well.

20 squats – key for your quads, core, and butt! Feet should width apart, back straight, and core engaged. Enjoy!

– Smile and do yoga! Simply breathe with a guided meditation.

Today's thoughts...

Stop comparing. Stop comparing yourself to friends, strangers, and previous versions of yourself. Comparing is a game that nobody wins. We are all worthy. Our being alive, being present in this world, gives us an inherent worthiness that can never be diminished or taken from us. Comparing is a vicious cycle, as it always means we are viewing someone or something as lesser and usually, it's hard not to feel we are the lesser! Let's make every effort to move away from that pattern of thought. It can never be a positive, growing experience. There is enough abundance in the universe. No one has to be the lesser. Support your friends, who are trying to succeed and grow and know that you deserve the same unconditional backing, whether others know how to give it to you or not. And, when anyone you know has a triumph in any area of life, celebrate with them! Be part of the exhilaration of somebody else's accomplishments. Blessings are contagious: be there for them and they will, in return, be there for you. We have this mistaken belief that there are limits in life – limits to joy, happiness, love, abundance, and prosperity, to whatever! These limiting beliefs make us feel that when someone else experiences success in some area of their life, it somehow diminishes or takes away from the potential for us to experience that same triumph. I just want to let you know that there is a limitless supply in the universe and there are no limits on what you seek. Set your intentions and put it out there! The more we celebrate the victories and triumphs of others, the more we will receive.

However you feel about yourself today and whether or not you believe you deserve it, make a commitment of taking care of yourself, as you are right now. Savour the time you spend with the people that matter and on the parts of your life that bring you the most happiness. There is no need to compare yourself to anybody else, because you are one of a kind. Other people have every right to be beautiful, prosperous, powerful, madly in love, or mildly in ecstasy. So, do you!

Word for today: JOY

Worry never robs tomorrow of its sorrow, it only saps today of its joy.

– Leo Buscaglia

Don't postpone joy until you have learned all of your lessons. Joy is your lesson.

— Alan Cohen

Joy is an essential spiritual practice, growing out of faith, grace, gratitude, hope, and love. It is the pure and simple delight in being alive. Joy is our elated response to feelings of happiness, experiences of pleasure, and awareness of abundance. It is, also, the deep satisfaction we know when we are able to serve others and be glad for their good fortune

Affirmation: I now seek to find joy in all things life has given me.

Exercise: Explore how joy can be found, even in the face of adversity.

_____

_____

_____

_____

_____

_____

_____

_____

_____

_____

_____

_____

_____

_____

SATURDAY

It's week four. You know the drill! Take the time today to go back to a day you may have missed or do something else you love to do, or maybe go crazy and try something you've always longed to do! Just, be kind to you. You are so lovely and wonderful. Enjoy the peace a guided meditation brings.

New Beginnings

New Beginnings

Wow! Four weeks have passed. Now, it's time to take a moment to reflect on your journey. Thank you for including me. I am truly honoured. If you have followed the program perfectly for the four weeks, that's incredible. You will undoubtedly feel stronger, healthier, and more empowered. If you have struggled to stay with the program and have done only bits and pieces, that's okay. Hopefully, that will be enough for you to know that it's worth the effort and more importantly, that you are worth the time and effort. We all struggle. There is no pass or fail. Please, do not stress and simply allow yourself the freedom to make a clean start, and try the program again from the beginning.

As you look back and notice how much or little of the program you were able to stay with, celebrate all you have learned. What stood out as an important turning point and how has that affected your life? Are you any clearer in the understanding that you direct your life and have the power to turn your stress into bliss? This is a huge learning and in time, you will come to know that it is a blessing. For fun, take the Simple Bliss Test again and look at your score. Is it higher than it was at the beginning?

My hope is that you have been able to make a difference in your life, over the past four weeks. So, where do you go now? What do you want to build into your life that will continue to support you in creating the reality you want? If you want to create more bliss and less stress in your life in the future, you need to set up your life in ways that will support this intention. What aspects of mind, body, and spirit have created the space to be able to bring more joy into your life? It is not easy to live your life mindfully. It is much easier to just react to situations as they come up. It's easier to be the victim of circumstance than to choose the path that will make a positive difference. Taking time daily to care for one-self, give yourself breathing space to allow yourself to remember what it is you really want and what you need to do, in order to continue in that desired direction. This way of being takes awareness, patience, compassion, understanding, love, and courage.

Some people believe that courage means facing ordeals without fear or resistance; like, the warrior going into battle. In truth, the real hero, the real warrior, is not the one without fear and resistance, but the one who has fear and resistance, acknowledges it, and goes for it, anyway. Even, when we are committed to change our lives and live more fully, we will still experience resistance and fear somewhere, along the way. That's normal and that is okay. Knowing what to do, when you encounter resistance and fear is going to serve you on your journey of recovery and beyond. If you acknowledge your triggers and stressors and are committed to the new path you are presently on, you will be able to dig deep and access the skills you have practiced in the last four weeks.

Developing a life of wellness means committing to your life's journey in its entirety, including, a spiritual practice. Our physical and spiritual yoga practice reminds us that there is no quick fix; it's about developing a deep and meaningful relationship with oneself and others, through the trials and joys of life. This is why in yoga, the setting of our intention is so vital. The intention of our yoga practice is to become a more peaceful, happy, and joyful person. Aren't these the essential qualities needed to support a renewed life in recovery? The necessary work that leads to this result becomes evident through our mind, body, and spirit practice. The areas we need to explore and go deeper are revealed through the physical and spiritual practices.

But, here's the thing, most social conditioning is built around the belief that it is possible to live in a pain-free, quick solution, immediate satisfactory environment. Unfortunately, we are rarely taught how to develop the tools to deal with the realities of life, with the struggles, and the challenges.

Wellness and recovery are not about getting rid of all of the challenges we face or by ignoring them, or controlling our environment. It's about keeping our peace of mind and sense of self, regardless of whether you experience ease and flow or stuckness and difficulties.

This is why it's crucial that you get the clarity you need and the resolve required to act on your triggers and stressors, before they take you somewhere you don't want to be. Understanding the true value of happiness as opposed to fleeting pleasure, cultivating an awareness of where we are at in the moment, and recognizing we have the power to choose. These are the valuable learnings in this program that will support your intentions of being present and living a life of wellness. It's a very different approach to life than what many of us know or have been taught to follow. It is an ongoing journey to deeper levels of knowledge and awareness, and happiness. It is a journey that requires courage, commitment, self-generated power, and above all, the recognition within ourselves, that we are unique and wonderful human beings. It is the journey of self-worthiness. It is the journey to you, without barriers or distractions, to the Spirit within you, your true Self, your Divine self.

You are worthy! You have made it here for a purpose. It is no accident that you have survived, against the odds, to be reading this seriously. You are a miracle! Never forget that. There is light within you!

God bless you and Namaste,
Carrie.

Yoga Postures

I thought it might be helpful to include a breakdown of the yoga postures you will be doing with me. For some of you, this might be old hat. But, for others, yoga is a new thing that you don't have much experience with. Keep an open mind and please, be patient with yourself. Don't be surprised, if the postures or positions are not comfortable, at first. You should feel your muscles lengthening and stretching gently, but it shouldn't be painful. If it is painful, ease up just a little. One of my yoga teachers, Eoin Finn of Blissology, has a great line, "Yoga postures are like a good relationship; always challenging, but never painful and they always make us grow!"

167

What is wonderful about yoga is that, you make it your own. Yoga demands that you listen to your body. And, hey, if you haven't been physically active, it is so normal that you will be tight, inflexible, and most likely sore, once you begin. Think of the soreness, as your muscles say *hello*. Having sore muscles is normal and I would encourage you not to stop the program because of it. You will work through this phase.

As you continue to practice, you will see your postures deepen. Perhaps, initially, you need to come out of Warrior II, before we move on. With time, you will develop the strength and ability to follow along. Please, don't get discouraged. Yoga is not about competition. It will meet you wherever you are presently. Know, that you can always come out of postures and then, resume. Begin with bent knees, whatever works for you. And, please, be realistic about where your body is. You may not have flexibility today, but with time, you will. Be kind to yourself and your body. The fact that you are here, showing up, is such a beautiful display of your strength and courage! Yes!

I would encourage you to get a yoga mat. Wear comfortable clothing that allows you to move. Remember, do what is right for you. Don't worry, if your leg is bent. You can't stretch deeply. Just show up and be present. In yoga, there is no judgment, no competition, and no expectations.

YOGA POSTURES

Mountain Pose
– Start with your feet parallel and toes pointing forward. Bring the feet together and balance the weight of your body on the four points of your feet. Stand tall and proud, shoulders back, and relaxed with arms extended downward, hands by your side.

Warrior One
– From Mountain pose, take a one foot medium stance back, turning the foot outward to the side. Adjust the positioning of the feet to allow your hips to be

"square" or both facing forward. Inhale, both arms straight overhead. Gaze is forward.

Warrior Two

- From Warrior I, open the back hip to face the side, turning the foot in the same direction. Your torso and hips should be facing the long edge of the mat. Arms extend front and back, at shoulder height. Gaze is forward.

Reverse Warrior

- From Warrior II, turn front hand, so palm faces skyward. Lower into the posture, while you bring the front hand skyward. Gaze is upward.

Triangle

- From Warrior II, straighten the front leg. Reach and extend the front arm, over the front leg. Begin to reach the front hand toward the leg as the torso turns upward, lengthening through the sides. Top hand reaches skyward.

Side Angle

- From Warrior II, place your front elbow on the front thigh as you extend your top arm skyward, revolving the torso with the motion of the hand.

Vinyasa

- A vinyasa is the sequence of movements that brings the yoga postures or asanas, together. The vinyasa begins in the lunge; moving into plank, lowering to chaturunga or low plank, inhaling to upward dog, and exhaling to downward dog.

Chaturunga

- Chaturunga is low plank. In yoga, the elbows are kept tucked in close to one's side body.

Downward Dog

- From all fours, tuck the toes under and extend the hips skyward. Legs and arms straight and extended. Feet and hands remain shoulder/hip width apart. Fingers are separated and the head is between the elbows. Extend down through the heels.

Upward Dog

- From low plank, chaturunga, straighten the arms and roll onto the tops of the feet. Legs are fully engaged and flexed. Knees and pelvis are off the ground. Roll the shoulders up and back. Gaze is forward or extending skyward.

Savasana

- Laying on your back, extend the arms and legs fully. Arms should be away from the body, palms facing upward. Allow the feel to drop open. This is also called Relaxation Pose.

Child's Pose

- From all fours, sink your hips down and back onto the heels. Extend the arms overhead. Relax on the ground or bring them around the back, around the sides of the body.

This should be a full relaxation pose.

Namaste. Peace. Love. Bliss. Happiness, my offerings to you!

Simple Bliss Test

Take this test, before you begin your four week program and again, after you complete it. This test is not meant to be used as a scientific tool, but a fun way to give you an overall idea of the extent of the stress and bliss in your life.

Rate each item on a scale of zero to ten, in terms of how accurately it describes you. A zero would be 'Does not describe me at all', a five would be 'Sometimes describes me', and a ten would be 'Always describes me'.

1. I am a happy person.
2. I have a clear purpose in my life that I'm pleased about.
3. I am achieving what I want in my life.
4. The stress in my life is moderate to manageable.
5. I am patient and calm in times of struggle.
6. I take good care of my physical and emotional health.
7. My life is exciting and challenging.
8. I get pleasure regularly from helping others.
9. There are people in my life who love me and who I enjoy spending time with.
10. My work is meaningful to me and serves others.

Total score out of a possible 100: _____

Results: If you scored 0–30, you don't have a lot of bliss in your life and you're probably experiencing one or more symptoms of stress. If you scored 31–60, you could probably use more bliss in your life, but you may not notice you feel all that stresses you out. If you scored 61–100, spread the love!

About Me:

Wow! I suppose the most important thing to know about me, is that *Yoga Recovery – Mind, Body, Spirit* comes from a source of love with the intention of being of service to you. I feel blessed to have created this work and I am overwhelmed with gratitude for you allowing me to be with you on this journey.

God bless and Namaste.

And in the end the love you take is equal to the love you make…

– the Beatles